# Praise for *The Emotional Edge*

"This book caught me by surprise; not just another 'self-help book for the wounded,' *The Emotional Edge* feels like a practical new psychology that gives profound and specific tools for the integration and healing of the Self. The processes, exercises, and meditations that Crystal Andrus Morissette provides are spot on! If applied, they will allow the reader to achieve a sense of inner peace and empowerment. A must-read!"

**—Sonia Choquette, *New York Times* bestselling author**

"For many years, Crystal Andrus Morissette has been a leader in the field of personal empowerment and motivation for women. She does it again with her new book, *The Emotional Edge*. If you'd like to get out from under the negative emotions that are holding you back, then this book shows you how. Congratulations, Crystal, on a beautiful job of reminding all women of their beauty and uniqueness."

**—Caroline Sutherland, author of *The Body Knows How to Stay Young***

"Crystal Andrus Morissette is an educator in the true sense of the word. She seeks to draw out of people, especially women, the best of them— their emotional, intellectual, and spiritual power, beauty, and truth. *The Emotional Edge* is a rare feast, one in which Ms. Morissette not only guides us to and through our own limits, fears, and beliefs, but one in which she walks alongside us, sharing her own story from denial and abuse to her own voice, truth, and purpose. The book begins with her earliest insight—'I just want to be empowered.' She has not only succeeded personally, but as a truly empowered human being, she inspires the rest of us to do the same. What is the essence of the truth she carries and transmits, 'We women are going to help heal the world.' Reward yourself by taking the journey of *The Emotional Edge*!"

**—David Bedrick, JD, author of *Talking Back to Dr. Phil:***
**  *Alternatives to Mainstream Psychology***

"After years of working with some of the most beautiful women in the world, I know firsthand there is a special energy or essence certain women embody. Crystal Andrus Morissette writes about it so perfectly in her powerful new book, *The Emotional Edge*. It's where true beauty comes from. But this book is about far more than just 'being beautiful.' It is designed to help every woman become the greatest expression of herself, to create her best life, to let go of beliefs and fears no longer serving her, and to know her true authentic self. *The Emotional Edge* is a must-read if you want to embody the beauty and strength of Woman Energy!"

**—Margot Boccia, A-list celebrity make-up artist**

# The Emotional Edge

DISCOVER YOUR INNER AGE,
IGNITE YOUR HIDDEN STRENGTHS,
AND REROUTE MISDIRECTED FEAR
TO LIVE YOUR FULLEST

## CRYSTAL ANDRUS MORISSETTE

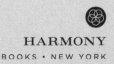

HARMONY

BOOKS · NEW YORK

Published in the United States by Harmony Books, an imprint of the
Crown Publishing Group, a division of Penguin Random House LLC, New York.
www.crownpublishing.com

Harmony Books is a registered trademark, and the Circle colophon is a
trademark of Penguin Random House LLC.

Library of Congress Cataloging-in-Publication Data
Andrus, Crystal, 1970–
    The emotional edge / Crystal Andrus.—First edition.
        pages    cm
  1.  Self-actualization (Psychology) in women.    2.  Self-realization in women.
3.  Emotions.    4.  Success.    I.  Title.
    BF637.S4A635 2015
    155.3'339—dc23

                                                                2015017956

ISBN 978-0-553-41842-2
eBook ISBN 978-0-553-41843-9

Printed in the United States of America

Book design by Debbie Glasserman
Illustrations by Kamen Nikolov
Jacket photograph by Vicky Drosos/Ikon Images/Getty Images

10 9 8 7 6 5 4 3 2 1

First Edition

I'm damned if I do and
I'm damned if I don't!
*So . . . what do I do?*

# Contents

# The
# Emotional
# Edge

# Introduction

I recently found my first journal. I flipped to the first page and read the first line:

*"I just want to be empowered."*

I wrote that on February 23, 1997. I was twenty-six years old. At the time, I was living in a lovely, panoramic house on the water with two beautiful, healthy daughters and a body-builder husband who came home every night. We owned a prosperous local health club, had money in the bank, and were investing monthly. I'd competed in and won fitness competitions such as the Junior Ontario Bodybuilding Championship and the Ms. Galaxy. I'd even set some regional track-and-field records and received the Mayor's Fitness Award. I'd managed a chain of health and racquetball clubs, including opening my own Crystal's Health & Fitness Spa when I was only twenty-two. I helped my husband open his Adonis Health & Fitness a year later. I had filmed a national episode of *Really Me* on YTV, on which I showed teenagers the power that exercise gave to me (for over five years it would run almost weekly across Canada); I'd been on the cover of a few fitness magazines; I'd been invited to be a guest on a national Canadian TV talk show (I said yes); and I'd been asked to pose in *Playboy* (I said no). I was attractive, strong, smart, kind, and friendly. I had everything: stainless steel professional series appliances, a six-hundred-square-foot kitchen, a table that sat twelve, a Corvette convertible in the garage, and a minivan.

What else could one want? And yet I didn't feel empowered. To me, empowerment meant feeling at ease within and about myself. And since I had *one idea* that dominated my thoughts—constantly reminding me of how unacceptable I was—I knew that, deep down, I wasn't empowered. Instead, I felt like maybe if I did more, I'd be more; if I got enough, I'd be enough. But I was tired of doing and having. And I was only twenty-six.

The night before I bought that blank journal, with my two-year-old sleeping peacefully in her canopy bed, I sat in my rocking chair nursing my youngest daughter and listening to Bob Greene's *Make the Connection*. My husband wasn't home from work yet. It was eleven p.m. I was crying. Sobbing, actually.

I'd hear Oprah say years later: "I didn't *really* know what the connection was that Bob was always talking about." That night, I didn't really know, either. But something in my heart cracked open just wide enough for me to believe that maybe I, too, could be happy and *thin again*.

As I look back, it shocks me that I wasn't thinking about finally dealing with the time when I was twelve years old and my father told me he was going out to buy a gallon of milk and a pack of cigarettes and then never came home. I'd had no idea my parents were even arguing, and yet nothing in my life would ever be the same again. My parents never once sat us down and explained what was happening. It was just never talked about. Dad moved in (three cities away) with his new, crazy girlfriend; and a month later, my older brother followed. I never said good-bye to either of them. I wasn't thinking about healing from the multitude of traumas that came after that—when my mother threw herself into bodybuilding and partying, moved her 24-year-old boyfriend in, or when the sexual abuse began to occur nightly. I rarely thought about how she kicked me out when I was fifteen, or how afraid I was that—despite the treatment I'd undergone for the early signs of cervical cancer when I was only seventeen, taking the city bus to the hospital by myself—*the cancer might come back again.*

*Nope.* I wasn't thinking about any of these things. I was thinking about my weight, specifically, How had *I* gotten *this* fat?

When I look back on that moment, I can see how completely lost I really was. I couldn't see that the suffering I was experiencing had nothing to do with numbers on a scale. Yet rather than face and begin to process the emotional, sexual, and physical abuse I'd suffered, I believed at that time that if I could just lose weight then I would be happy.

We've all been consumed with disempowered, repetitive thoughts—misdirected fear—the stuff that distracts and numbs us from the real stuff.

Skip ahead to nine years later: 2006.

I remember the bewildering feeling I had when I walked into the largest bookstore in Canada—Chapters Indigo at Toronto Eaton Centre, in the heart of downtown—and there was my face, front and center in the store, blown up on huge posters as the "Reader's Choice"!

With stacks and stacks of my books placed on tables at the front of the store, I picked up the little brochure that explained the poll and read my name in print, there among a list of people who were changing the world:

> To create our list, we asked over 40,000 irewards members to recommend the books that helped them lead a healthier lifestyle and achieve their personal best.
>
> CHAPTERS | INDIGO | COLES

Forty thousand readers were polled across Canada to see which book had most influenced their life and that first little journal, *Simply . . . Woman! The 12-Week Body-Mind-Soul Total Transformation Program* came in at number fourteen! I was in complete and utter shock. How on earth did little ole *me*, who initially *self*-published my little ole journal, achieve this kind of recognition?

I continued to scan down the list of names below mine: Julia Cameron, Dr. Phil, Harvey Diamond, Anthony Robbins, Don Miguel Ruiz, Joel Osteen, Robin Sharma, Neale Donald Walsch, Dalai Lama, Eckhart Tolle, John Gray, Andrew Weil, Sean Covey, Clarissa Pinkola Estés, Jack Canfield, and M. Scott Peck. I was even ahead of one of my mentors and first publisher: Louise L. Hay.

I was amazed! This success affirmed to me that no matter who you are or what has happened to you, if you decide to, you can create a successful life! I knew, in that moment, that empowerment is our birthright! We were designed to expand our lives! To follow what "lights" us up and to let our "inner light" expand into the brightest, happiest, most empowered version of ourselves possible.

In fact, science tells us that we live in an infinite, ever-expanding universe and that we are a part of that universe. Stephen Hawking explains it in *A Brief History of Time*:

> The discovery that the universe is expanding was one of the greatest intellectual revolutions of the twentieth century. With hindsight, it is easy to wonder why no one had thought of it before. Newton, and others, should have realized that a static universe would soon start to contract under gravity. But suppose instead that the universe is expanding. If it was expanding fairly slowly, the force of gravity would cause it to stop expanding and then to start contracting. However, if it was expanding at more than a critical rate, gravity would never be strong enough to stop it, and the universe would continue forever. This is a bit like what happens when one fires a rocket upward from the surface of the earth. If it has a fairly slow speed, gravity will eventually stop the rocket and it will start falling back. On the other hand, if the rocket has more than a certain critical speed (about seven miles per second), gravity will not be strong enough to pull it back, so it will keep going away from the earth forever.

When someone takes away your ability to expand your own life, you are oppressed, controlled, and disempowered. You begin, as Hawking points out, to "contract," that is, to shrivel and die. But when you are your own person, able to make your own decisions and follow your dreams, you can expand yourself and your abilities infinitely. Your desires and passions are similar to the rocket firing upward from the surface of this earth. If they are powerful enough, gravity will not be strong enough to pull them back. This, in turn, expands the world around you. Your dreams manifest!

The necessity of choice is why all our religious texts insist that God gave us "free will." We must be able to make our own decisions in order to expand consciousness—to be empowered!

> When you take away choice, you take away empowerment. When you think you have no choice, you disempower yourself.

As you take back the reins in your life by focusing on expansion, you, too, expand the collective consciousness. Empowered people are in alignment with the universe. Suffering arrives to show us where we are out of alignment. But we can't give what we don't have.

To give you a simple metaphor of expansion: Take a deep, fully expanded breath and notice how you feel. Hold for a second. Now, contract your lungs and exhale completely. Notice the difference in your body, posture, and confidence between the two.

Now, try taking another deep breath . . . but this time, hold it for five seconds. Then, take three more tiny inhales and hold them, too. Notice how holding on begins to suffocate you.

Finally, blow all the air out of your lungs and hold your breath again. Quickly exhale three extra puffs. Hold. Stay static. Don't move. Don't breathe. Don't expand. Wait . . .

Fear constricts, contracts, and holds on. Gripping. Almost panicked. Life or empowerment, on the other hand, trusts the gentle inhale that will follow. Receiving. Releasing. Allowing. Expanding.

> We can't expand and empower collective consciousness until we expand and empower our own personal consciousness.

The purpose of this book is to empower you to expand your life so you can become the greatest expression of you possible—to give you the Emotional Edge! A big part of this comes from understanding your Emotional Age and how you are showing up in the world. We will dig into your Emotional Age in Chapter One.

Once you get the Emotional Edge, you'll never give your power away again without recognizing it. You'll see when you're sabotaging yourself and come to understand why. You'll be able to detect when you're around other people who are attempting to take your power from you and you will learn how to protect, support, and nurture yourself. You will begin to live in a world that is expanding to enable your wildest dreams, hopes, and ambitions to become realities.

*The Edge* is twofold: it is a powerful, penetrating, expansive quality—the horizon line of possibilities—that creates freedom, happiness, liberation, self-assuredness, and power; it is also the place on "your own path" where you are able to thrive as an individual while joyously honoring the commitments you've made to those you care about. You are able to channel your fear and anger into courage and willingness. You are able to live your best life without guilt, shame, or blame.

There are hidden rules we must learn if we want to feel empowered. The Emotional Edge shares these rules so that no more will you feel like a victim of circumstance, genetics, or your past.

Every experience you have colors the way you relate to the world. Your life isn't necessarily shaped by the things you've spent the most time doing or the people you've spent the most time with; powerful emotional experiences can happen in a flash but leave an indelible mark. The Emotional Edge will not only help you identify the events that have defined your life, it will also prepare you to be better equipped to deal with the future. It will help you seek out experiences that will fill your life with joy and strength, and steel you against experiences that might otherwise pull you down.

This book is about acknowledging, feeling, healing, letting go, and moving beyond. It's about dealing with the ways people have disappointed, hurt, or misled you, and coming through these emotions on the other side stronger, maybe even invincible!

The Emotional Edge is about identifying what is standing between you and your most empowered Emotional Age; together we will face these roadblocks and overcome them. The bottom line is that life is not what happens to you, it's what you *do* with what happens to you.

Although this book is nongender and many men and couples will benefit from reading it, I personally wrote it for every woman who is tired of thinking about her flaws, fears, failures, and *fat*—those disempowered repetitive thoughts that are preventing you from becoming your greatest Self.

Women, in particular, struggle with Empowered Communication. For thousands and thousands of years, women have been oppressed. Most of our mothers, grandmothers, and all of our great-great-grandmothers were unable to vote, hold office, own property, speak out publicly, or have any rights over their own bodies. It has been only in the last few generations that women were even considered a "person" by law.

Here in North America where I live, Canada was the first country to grant women the status of "person" in 1917; the United States followed in 1920. Prior to that, the word *person* referred only to men. A British common law ruling from 1867 emphasized, "Women are persons in matters of pains and penalties but are not persons in matters of rights and privileges." We were possessions of our fathers, passed down to our husbands. We've been "groomed" for disempowerment for thousands of years.

Over the last fifty years, the world has radically changed—from radio to television to computers and Internet. We have thousands of channels to surf now, pornography at our fingertips, chat rooms to consume us, and dating services to supply our never-ending demand. We have toys, gadgets, devices, and systems. We have wireless, cellular, satellite lives with two incomes, two cars in the driveway, and a TV in every room. And yet, with all this stuff, we're lonelier than we can possibly explain. We're so full that we're empty.

Feminism was not intended to cause the breakdown of the "American family," even if it did. It was meant to give women their rights to become empowered . . . to expand their Emotional Edges! The same way men are able to!

The problem is that many women still struggle with knowing their worth. Even in the year 2015, when a little girl is born, she is a "Miss." If she should be so lucky as to get married, she becomes a "Mrs." If she gets divorced or never marries, her title shifts to the stern-sounding "Ms."

Boys, on the other hand, are born a "Mr." and die a "Mr." Their identity is completely separate and untouched by the women in their lives.

At the Vancouver Peace Summit 2009, the Dalai Lama said, "The Western woman will heal the world." I believe him. Not because the Western woman is smarter, better, or more enlightened than other women, but because today we have the ability to expand our Emotional Edges further than ever before and further than many women around the world are able to even today; women who have no rights or personal freedoms; who can't drive a vehicle or pursue an education. The Western woman can chase her dreams, follow her heart, and make her own decisions. She has more options and more choices, which means more empowerment. You simply can't have half the population oppressed and ever expect to find world peace.

The truth is, men and women are different. We all know this. In the Western world, many women have tried to become more masculine to fit into the workplace climate—a place where we were not allowed to be prior to the last fifty years. I believe it is time to celebrate and encourage our differences and allow our two genders to come together—masculine and feminine—to create the balance this world desperately needs.

Although we can't turn back time (nor should we), we can reflect on years gone by—on what worked and what didn't—and learn how to do things better in the future, starting right now! We can create a new "Love Language." (We'll talk more about this in Chapter Seven.)

Women—*worldwide*—desire compassion, fairness, kindness, honesty, love, joy, and peace of mind in our relationships—personal and professional. The rest of the world is watching how the "empowerment of the Western woman" is working for society. The goal is for our empowerment to spill over to women in third-world, communist, and patriarchal countries.

In 2015, Phumzile Mlambo-Ngcuka, executive director of

UN Women, was quoted as saying: "A girl born this year will be eighty before she lives in a world of gender equality."

**We must Close the Gap faster.**
**#CloseTheGap**

In the meantime, there are still millions of women—babies, daughters, sisters, aunties, mothers, and grandmothers—around the world who need our help. Women who, even now, are considered nothing more than a domestic commodity and a birthing machine; women who can't vote, study, or own property; who have a voice but can't use it; who are controlled, coerced, hurt, abused, manipulated, and exploited and who want nothing more than to be free . . . women who would be severely reprimanded if they did half of what I do. I guarantee that in a different century, I would have been burned at the stake.

As Caitlin Moran writes in the shockingly bold, runaway bestseller *How to Be a Woman*, "It's been a long, slow 100,000-year trudge out of patriarchy. There are still parts of the world where women are not allowed to touch food when they're menstruating or are socially ostracized for failing to give birth to boys. Even in America and Europe, women are still so woefully underrepresented in everything—science, politics, art, business, space travel . . ."

# The Woman Matters

So much has already been written about the Mother and the Child Archetypes, as well as Carl Jung's the Father, the Wise Old Man, and the Hero—but what about the archetype the Woman?

*Is there one?*

And if so, has it been around long enough to give our mind an immediate message that requires no further explanation the way Mother does?

In fact, the Woman Archetype is something relatively new in human history. Even for the brilliant psychologist Carl Jung, his most evolved archetype when it comes to women is the Wise Old Woman.

Jungian psychoanalyst Dr. Clarissa Pinkola Estés has written extensively about female archetypes and has even recorded an entire audio series on the Dangerous Old Woman. Even Joseph Campbell's *Hero's Journey* refers to only male archetypes. But what about the rest of us—the wise twenty-, thirty-, forty-, fifty-, or even, sixty-something-year-old woman? What about the Shero?

**What do you think of when you hear the word *woman*? Who is she? What is her archetype?**

Since the beginning of time there were mothers and daughters in human communities. Their role and the core of what they stand for haven't changed.

Mother represents safety, responsibility, and protection—mature, self-sacrificing, and perhaps even boring. Daughter conjures up helpless, cute, immature, and, often, flighty or flakey—irresponsible.

But what do we think when we speak the word *woman*? Has her role and the core of what she stands for changed? How would a woman manage her life, deal with challenges, teach people how to treat her, and take care of herself? Is she spiritual and sexy? Is she thin, voluptuous, fit, or fat? Or do her size and shape not matter?

Can she be prosperous and independent, or does a woman need a man? Does she need sex and attention, or does she need no one? And what happens if a woman has children? Must she become saintly, selfless, and self-abnegating?

This book is, in part, an attempt to define what being an empowered woman means, *and the answer to this will serve men, too*! It is time for women to stop having to explain themselves, to justify their ambitions, to search fruitlessly for possibilities and role models. It's time for the word *woman* to become an archetype that requires no further explanation. It will be a clearly defined symbol.

On a personal note:

I teach empowerment because I needed to learn how to be empowered. I needed to see where and how I was contributing to the drama and dysfunction in my life.

I can see now that in my youth and even into my mid-thirties, I desperately struggled with setting boundaries and with saying no because I was never taught that I mattered and my needs mattered. A lack of parental support left me feeling worthless, while sexual abuse left me feeling tarnished—like used goods. In my mind, why did it matter now who touched, abused, or took advantage of me? Shame has this way of stripping away our dignity and self-respect.

Moving out of my mother's house at fifteen and couch surfing for three years taught me that I was alone in the world. I learned to trust no one, although I tried desperately to please everyone. Inevitably, I felt empty and lost, and most often I felt alone, unwanted, and unimportant. I just wanted to be happy and stay happy. I just wanted to be loved. I just wanted to be empowered.

I could get along with just about anyone (perhaps because I didn't let anyone get too close), and yet the most challenging relationships I had were with my immediate family members. Put us in a house together for a day, and you could count on at least one of us crying, one of us yelling, and one of us going home seething mad, determined never to speak to the others again! Ever! Period! Done! Over and out!

All I kept wondering was: *Can't we all just get along?*

But we couldn't just get along.

*Why?*

I knew it wasn't for a lack of love. We loved one another.

I knew it wasn't for a lack of brains. We were all smart.

We were all nice-looking, and yet being attractive didn't seem to help, either.

I knew it had nothing to do with inner strength. Everyone in my family had endured some kind of horrible experience— rape, molestation, abandonment; physical, verbal, sexual, and/or emotional abuse; addiction; betrayal and neglect— and yet we were all pretty fearless in our independent lives. So I crossed out weakness as the reason why we couldn't get along.

We had the cars, trinkets, houses, and watches. Rolex was a household name in my family. Our homes were immaculate, our cars shone, our yards looked like golf courses, and our clothes were smartly pressed. But looking perfect didn't help us get along, either!

I'd hear from others how fabulous certain members of my family were, and yet we were so *un*fabulous with one another. I'm sure they all felt the same way.

So *why* couldn't we consistently communicate our needs in a clear, honest, and peaceful way with one another? Why couldn't we each give and receive and stay in a place of harmony, happiness, and well-being?

Why couldn't a smart, successful, savvy group of people who essentially loved one another treat one another better?

> I had to figure it out. I knew the answers lay somewhere inside of me. It was an inside job.

Sure—the people in my life had plenty to do with my chaos. But I innately knew they were merely showing up to reveal my unhealed stories—*my suffering*—to me.

Triggers, I know now, are gifts to show us that we are suffering. They tell us that we need a healing of the heart and a shift in our mind-set. Triggers let us know that we need to recontextualize our "stories" to lift us to higher ground emotionally. I innately knew all the arguing had something to do with our Emotional Age and how we were showing up in the world and in our family's dynamics. We kept bringing out the worst in one another. Never-ending fighting and undermining.

I won't lie: asking for the answers to these questions spiraled me down the rabbit's hole. And there was no going back. Once I accepted the initial answers that I'd asked for, I received more than I could imagine *and then some*.

Writing this book felt like teeter tottering into no-man's-land; I was afraid to move forward but more afraid to go back. The vulnerability I felt sharing my own truths, mixed with the audacity of writing a book about how to heal your own wounds and become a stronger, striving person, both terrified and electrified me. There is a fine line between madness and mystic. After many Dark Nights of the Soul, I've discovered my truth: Love Heals Everything. Every. Thing.

Freedom is on the other side of *The Emotional Edge*.

Turn off the lights and come away with me . . .
Warmly,

Crystal Andrus Morissette

There is a force in the Universe, which, if we permit it, will flow through us and produce miraculous results.

MAHATMA GANDHI

# CHAPTER ONE

# Your Emotional Age

## "REMEMBER"

Emancipate yourselves from mental slavery.
None but ourselves can free our mind . . .

BOB MARLEY + THE WAILERS

Most of us have heard about Biological Age. It is a scientific concept that measures how well, or badly, your body is functioning relative to your Chronological Age. For example, you may be sixty years old but you've eaten well, exercised, drunk plenty of clean water, minimized stress, and so on. Your body might be functioning as well as someone twenty years younger than you as a result of your self-care. We've also heard stories about thirty-year-olds who have lived too hard and recklessly, leaving themselves with bodies and hearts that bear extra decades' worth of scars.

Emotional Age is a similar concept to Biological Age. But rather than predicting how young or old our physical bodies are, Emotional Age helps us understand how empowered or disempowered we are emotionally.

It helps explain how we've been communicating, compromising, socializing, and interacting with others. For example, we've all seen those sixty-plus-year-old persons who, regardless of their chronological age, behave like angry teenagers when they're upset—yelling, screaming, slamming doors, and stonewalling. Conversely, we've also witnessed the young, twentysomething-year-olds who carry the weight of the world on their shoulders, acting way too mature for their age, silently burdening not only their own worries and fears but taking on those of their loved ones, as well.

We've also seen the older guys with young trophy wives, and immediately we know these men are father figures, in a "parental role," while the young women are operating as children, in the "daughter archetype."

In other words, we all innately recognize when people are acting outside of their Emotional Age; we've just never given it a name *until now*!

Emotional Age is different from being an "old soul" or a "young soul." It has little to do with Intelligence Quotient, Emotional Intelligence, or economic or social status, and it has *everything* to do with the way we act and react to life.

**The more empowered our Emotional Age, the better our lives will be!**

The purpose of this book is to be a shortcut for the reader—a condensed, ready-to-use life stratagem or practical psychology based on Emotional Age. It offers a communication style, scale, and strategy called the Empowerment Spectrum that will provide readers with an edge or an advantage in all their relationships.

## The Empowerment Spectrum

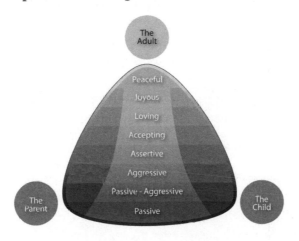

The Empowerment Spectrum outlines the concept of our identities being formed by a combination of three Dominant Emotional Archetypes—the Child, the Parent, the Adult. Within these three archetypes, we communicate on a scale from passive (disempowered) to peaceful (empowered).

For years leading up to writing this book, I'd half-jokingly refer to these three Dominant Emotional Archetypes as my "Mother Energy," "Daughter Energy," and "Woman Energy." The interesting thing was how everyone seemed to understand what I meant when I used these terms. They seemed universal—as if everyone had these same three personas that ran their lives, too.

The Parent Archetype is the selfless part of us that gives, protects, and serves. It is the archetype that drives us to sacrifice our own needs for the needs of others.

The Child Archetype is the selfish part of us that wants, takes, and desires. Fearful and gripping, this archetype drives us to take care of our own needs before the needs of others.

The Adult Archetype is the integration and transcendence of the noblest qualities of each of these two archetypes into the fully empowered Self. This is the archetype that balances the Self in a way that expands outward without losing connectedness inward.

Without realizing it, our behavior is usually dictated by one of these Three Dominant Archetypes, depending upon the person we're dealing with; often one of these archetypes will dominant most aspects of our life.

Eric Berne, founder of Transactional Analysis, talked extensively about people having a life script that they begin to "mentally write" from a very young age. In *What Do You Say After You Say Hello*, he states:

> Each person decides in early childhood how he will live and how he will die, and that plan, which he carries in his head wherever he goes, is called a script. His trivial behavior may be decided by reason, but his important decisions are already made . . .

By the time you were five years old, you'd made decisions about how lovable and worthy you were, how best to survive in this world, and what life would give back to you. You developed a "story" in your childlike mind by watching and listening to your parents, aunts, uncles, grandparents, and siblings—and the emotional archetypes they embodied—and you accepted "your part" in the story of your family. Your Dominant Emotional Archetype is based on what you believe is the safest or smartest way of getting your needs met. In fact, immediately upon birth, you began writing your survival story, which formed your Dominant Emotional Archetype.

■ **This life script is the basis of Emotional Age.**

## Your Brilliant Brain

Here are the facts: Your brain doesn't work at random. One of its biggest objectives is to ensure your existence. Your brain is far more concerned with your physical or emotional survival than it is with presenting you an objective reality.

Cognitive neuroscientist Michael Gazzaniga, who founded the Centers for Cognitive Neuroscience at the University of California, Davis, and at Dartmouth College, suggests that one of the functions of the left hemisphere of our brain is to become an Interpreter. His research shows that as early as infancy our brain is prone to making up a story about who we are—a narrative upon which our identity is based.

Psychologist and science historian Michael Shermer, author of *The Believing Brain*, describes it this way:

> The brain is a belief engine. From sensory data flowing in through the senses, the brain naturally begins to look for and find patterns, and then infuses those patterns with meaning . . . These meaningful patterns become beliefs, and these beliefs shape our understanding of reality.

In a way, your "story" makes decision making easier because it tells you who you need to be in order to best survive in this world. The reason why your brain does this is one of adaptation. The problem is, your life script can be based on lies.

For example, if the environment you grew up in convinced you that steadiness and reliability were necessary traits, that you must take care of the people you most love, that you need to be "a good little girl or boy" in order to be safe, then you will become the Parent Archetype in front of the world. Neglecting yourself for the sake of others becomes your best form of protection, even if it robs you of safety, freedom, and happiness!

If, on the other hand, your environment sent messages that you were at the mercy of the people in the power seat, that your needs would be met only if you could ingratiate yourself with the right people, that being charming, helpless, difficult, or demanding was the safest way to get by, you will remain the Child Archetype.

Our Interpreter creates a story about how *the world* wants us to be. The purpose of this life script is to have a shorthand for what keeps us safe—this way, in moments when we need to make split decisions, we have a mental shortcut that instantly tells us how to choose! But of course these stories hurt us as much as, or more than, they help us.

*It reminds me of the powerful true story of the seven-hundred-year-old clay Buddha from Thailand:*

In 1957, a group of Buddhist monks were moving a five-ton statue of a clay Buddha that had sat in a deserted temple for hundreds of years. In the midst of moving it, the straps broke and the statue fell to the ground. The horror of the monks soon turned to surprise when one of them noticed something glistening below the cracked clay. After running to get a chisel, one monk began to chip away at the statue (which would have taken a lot of courage), and revealed a solid Golden Buddha underneath the clay.

The story goes that hundreds of years earlier, when the Burmese army was entering Thailand, the monks at the time knew that the solid-gold statue would be stolen, so they devised a plan: cover it in clay so it wouldn't be deemed as valuable.

The plan worked.

The trouble was, every monk was murdered by the army, so the tale could never be passed on . . . until the statue was finally safe enough.

*Safe enough . . .*

The story of the sacred Golden Buddha is a perfect analogy for why we choose a Dominant Emotional Archetype to hide behind. It becomes our clay. Our protection. Our mask.

The good news is your gold can never be stolen. It can be buried—perhaps so deeply that you think it's not there—but never lost.

Take a moment and think back to when you were a child, when you were golden and you knew it!

> **Why wouldn't the world love you?**
> **Why couldn't you shine bright?**
> **Why wouldn't you be safe?**

*But things happened . . .*

Maybe the people in your life didn't realize how brilliant, gorgeous, talented, and fabulous you were, and by the time you were a young adult, you'd made some survival-like decisions: Cover my talents, dreams, needs, and desires. Cover my potential. Cover my gold. Tuck it away until I'm safe enough to shine bright . . . and keep it safe enough in the meantime.

When you were little—boy or girl—your internal guidance system (your personal GPS) was in pristine working order. You trusted yourself! You thought for yourself! You believed in yourself! You had a mind of your own! You knew exactly what you wanted and what you liked! You were empowered! You were happy! You knew when you were hungry, full, tired, and satisfied! You never second-guessed yourself! It didn't occur to you *not* to like yourself!

As you grew, you were taught *not* to trust your feelings. Maybe you were told such things as "little girls are sugar and spice and everything nice, and little boys are snips and snails and puppy-dog tails." Maybe you were taught to wipe that smile off your face, to respect authority, that children are to be seen and not heard, and to eat all the food on your plate (there are starving people in the world), only to be judged later if you started looking chubby?

Maybe you were told to stop crying and to put a smile *back* on your face, and that if you don't have anything nice to say, don't say anything at all? Maybe your siblings were mean to, abusive to, or neglectful of you? Perhaps you had teachers, grandparents, aunts, uncles, even neighborhood kids who bullied or teased you?

The list of the ways disempowered people put "their stuff" on us is long. In the end, most of us were taught to resist our own feelings, not to judge a book by its cover (meaning "don't trust your instincts"), and don't rock the boat.

A part of what we will do together in the coming chapters is recontextualize your past so that you can find the lessons—or the gift in the garbage, so to speak—that will enable you to clean up your unfinished business and heal the old wounds.

Bear in mind, understanding your past doesn't mean you will know your Self any better. It simply means you will know more *about* yourself. Knowing your *true* Self is a much easier process than you can imagine. We will do this together!

It is also important you know that adversity does not show you who you *really* are; it shows you where you are *not* in alignment with your Real Self. It shows you where you are not in alignment with the laws of the universe, where you are going against the flow. Adversity shows you where you are in resistance to your own empowerment. It shows you the lies you've bought into, the stories you've created, and how you've gotten so caught up in the drama that you're unsure how to escape it. The thing to keep in mind is that this is all happening unconsciously so there is no point in beating yourself up over it.

The question to ask now is, "Am I willing to look at why I would have created this life script or theme for my relationships?

The fact remains, suffering no longer serves me. It doesn't have to serve you, either. Suffering is not in alignment with the ever-expanding universe. Suffering constricts. Happiness expands. As Buddha said: "Pain is inevitable. Suffering is optional."

My promise to you is that this book will teach you how to let go of your suffering by showing you how to learn from your trials and tribulations and then take back your power. It will teach you simple mindfulness techniques so that you can catch yourself when you're about to fall into a Dominant Emotional Archetype that doesn't serve you. Most important, it will teach you the truth of who you really are.

We will use love, compassion, and kindness. Beating up on ourselves doesn't work. Denying our suffering doesn't either. So we're going to start telling ourselves the truth but we're going to surround it with a nice, soft cushion. Truth *without* love might be an effective teacher, but it is harsh, punishing, and can leave deep scars; truth *with* love heals rather than hurts and is far more effective in the long term.

The bottom line is that we all have a past. We can't keep running from it or looking back with fear and dread. We can turn our wounds into wisdom.

## What Did You Learn Growing Up?

In the book *Born to Win*, Muriel James and Dorothy Jongeward explain that our earliest interactions with our parents are crucial in determining our Dominant Emotional Archetype:

> Infants, almost as if they had radar, begin to pick up messages about themselves and their worth through their first experiences of being touched or being ignored by others. Soon they see facial expressions and respond to them as well as to touch and sounds. Children who are cuddled affectionately, smiled at, and talked to receive different messages from those who are handled with fright, hostility, or anxiety. Children who receive little touch and who experience parental indifference or hostility are discounted. They learn to feel they are not-OK and perhaps may feel like a "nothing."

Understanding our childhood script is the first step toward understanding the Emotional Age that we've chosen: children's first feelings about themselves are likely to remain the most powerful force in their life dramas, significantly influencing the psychological positions they take and the roles they play.

Our script, or survival story, has a structure very similar to that of a theatrical play. The script has acts that are broken into scenes filled with dialogue; it has plots that build to a climax. Like all good dramas, we also have a theme. This theme is the driving force behind the Emotional Age that guides us.

We create our character or decide on our Dominant Emotional Archetype based on our gender, culture, religious values, and family roles. We make decisions about life and ourselves based on the events we experienced and the beliefs we were taught. We do all of this because of the need to survive.

The biggest influence on your Emotional Age is what you learned from your parents—primarily your same-sex parent.

Take a moment and look back at your earliest memories. What did you learn about the following topics from your mother (if you're a woman) or from your dad (if you're a man)?

- Being a girl versus being a boy
- What it means to be a woman
- What it means to be a man
- Sex
- Love
- Marriage
- Fidelity and commitment
- Money
- Beauty, fashion, and social status
- Children
- Education
- Food, cooking, celebration
- God, superstition, and evil
- Independent thinking
- Expressing your feelings
- Your worth
- Your future
- Your looks
- Your brains
- Your *Self* . . . what did you learn about the greatest part of you?

If you take the time to sit quietly and answer each of the above questions, you might begin to understand where some of your notions about what's important came from. Whether you share those values or have worked hard to fight against them, you learned them from somewhere. Your brilliant brain retained the messages that were sent to you at a very formative age, and those have helped shape what you value and how you set your priorities.

As we each forged our own life script to determine how we respond to others, we asked ourselves three simple yet poignant questions:

1. Who Am I?
2. Who Are You?
3. What's My Purpose?

Throughout this book, we will examine these three questions. To begin with, I've created a short quiz to help you figure out which Emotional Age—or, more specifically, which Dominant Emotional Archetype—you've been using to navigate your life. It's important that you respond with the way you'd most likely handle the pretend scenarios described on the following several pages rather than how you'd prefer to react.

## Take the Quiz

Whether you're aware of it or not, each of us is on a life path, or trajectory, traveling toward an ultimate destiny. If you're honest with yourself, you can closely predict where you'll end up just by evaluating the choices you're making today. What many of us don't realize is that our choices, even the almost insignificant ones, are driven by the emotional state we're in.

Understanding where we resonate emotionally can mean the difference between living a life of joy, love, abundance, purpose, and passion and living a life of loneliness, frustration, inadequacy, and fear.

It's important you know that you are not your past. You are not constrained by your story, experiences, or even your current reality. You are not defined by your parents, religion, culture, or upbringing. If you knew who you *really* are, you'd be in awe of yourself—the same way millions of people stand in awe before the Golden Buddha statue in Bangkok.

Some of us may need to make some small tweaks to correct the course of our life path, while others will need a major overhaul in order to radically alter their trajectory. Either way, this book will help you understand how to make the necessary changes to create a life you love, but first it's important to understand which Emotional Age you've been using to navigate thus far.

Take the following quiz to learn your Emotional Age. There are no wrong answers here, no need to try to figure out how to respond in the most politically correct way. These are questions to help you better understand what is standing between you and the most vibrant, dynamic, invigorated life possible!

Along with this quiz, start paying attention to how you respond to any challenges that come your way. Remember that there are no wrong answers and no wrong way of behaving right now; just make an honest evaluation of how you respond to others in a variety of situations. If you are gentle and truthful with yourself, you'll quickly identify whether you're in an empowered Adult Archetype versus a Parent or Child Archetype.

Finally, if you really want more clarity in determining your

Emotional Age, ask the three people closest to you to take this quiz on your behalf. In other words, how do they feel you would handle the following scenarios? (You have to promise not to get upset with them for giving you their most honest answers.)

The objective of the Emotional Age Quiz is to help you see yourself more clearly so that you can better understand what makes you act the way you do. Once you see the truth of how you handle a variety of situations, you can make changes that will allow you to communicate and function more honestly.

The most important factor during this quiz is to be as honest as possible with yourself . . . about yourself . . . because this is for you! We can only change things we're willing to face. It's imperative you see the truth of the reality you're creating.

## EMOTIONAL AGE QUIZ

For each question, circle the answer that best represents your typical reaction or choice. (Please visit **www.TheEmotionalEdge .com** to take the interactive free quiz.):

1. If I look in the mirror and don't like what I see. I will:
    a. Stop looking. Appearances don't matter that much. Sure, I wish I looked better, but who has the time? It's not that important.
    b. Worry . . . maybe worry a lot. There's nothing wrong with wanting to look and feel my best. Keeping up my appearance is a constant pressure in my life. I'd certainly consider plastic surgery if I thought I needed it.
    c. Spend more time on self-care. If it's something I have control over (i.e., I could exercise more, eat more nutritiously, or get my hair styled), I make the necessary

changes. If it's something I have no control over, I love and accept myself as I am. I could be better. I could be worse.

2. My sixteen-year-old daughter comes home pregnant. I am:

   a. Sad, afraid, and even mortified. How could this happen? I feel like a failure as a parent. I know she needs my help. She is still a child herself.

   b. Angry. What was she thinking? I love her, but I certainly hope she doesn't expect me to take care of this baby. I can't handle this right now. I have too many problems of my own.

   c. Disappointed for her. Of course, this is not good timing: she's only sixteen! I will make sure she knows her options, and I'll support whatever decision she ultimately feels is right for *her* life.

3. I've found a new passion I want to turn into my own business. When I tell my family they laugh and remind me of some of my past ideas. I feel:

   a. Conflicted and suddenly unsure. What do I really know about running this kind of business? Maybe I need to focus on my family and the things currently working in my life.

   b. Hurt and defensive. My family is so negative and unsupportive. How could anyone become successful with a family like mine? They have always judged me harshly.

   c. A little disappointed but not deterred. Instead of "giving up" or "bottling my frustration" at my family's reaction, I keep pushing forward and try to see if I can take anything productive from their criticism.

4. My neighbor comes over while I'm fixing something on my brand-new, very expensive car. I don't ask for his help. He offers. But in the midst of fixing it, he slips and drops

a wrench, which dents the side of my car and chips the paint. I:

**a.** Insist that he need not worry about it. It was an accident. I'll absolutely pay for it. No worries!

**b.** Insist that he pay for it. This was his error, and it shouldn't be my problem. This could cause bad blood between neighbors if he doesn't pay up.

**c.** Insist that he need not worry about it. But I will never let him work on my vehicle again. A good guy but a sloppy guy! Just like the saying: Fool me once, shame on you. Fool me twice, shame on me.

**5.** For months, my boss has been pressuring me more and more to work harder, stay longer at the office, and cater to his personal needs (getting his lunch, bringing him coffee, buying gifts for his wife, etc.) by giving me his personal credit card. I feel:

**a.** Needed but exhausted. I appreciate his trust in me, but I'm feeling overwhelmed and perhaps even underpaid. But I don't want to rock the boat. I'm blessed to have this job, and I'm hoping that now he'll owe me support down the line.

**b.** Fed up. I'm debating about taking his credit card and buying myself my own little gifts for all the "extras" I do without pay, or soon telling him to stick this job up his #%*. I'm worth more than this.

**c.** Concerned. It's time to arrange a meeting with my boss to professionally explain my perspective and renegotiate either my remuneration or job responsibilities. I will have to find a way to do this within the next week. I won't let it drag on any longer.

**6.** If my lover/partner makes a negative comment about my body, I:

    **a.** Shrug it off and pretend it doesn't hurt. I don't want to appear too sensitive. My body could use some improving. I'm far from perfect. Besides, I know (s)he loves me.

    **b.** Quietly storm out of the room and sulk for a while. This just makes me feel worse about myself. Why can't I just look better? I'm so frustrated with myself. And how dare (s)he criticize my body? I will never forget his/her cruel words. Ever.

    **c.** I know the effort I put in to exercising regularly and eating healthily. There might be things I want to improve, but overall I'm happy with myself. If he/she continues to disrespect me, I won't stay in the relationship.

**7.** I run into an old high school friend and find out she's become wildly successful and looks like a million bucks. I feel:

    **a.** Happy for her. I could never achieve her accomplishments. What an amazing woman she is. I always knew she'd "make it."

    **b.** Conflicted and, perhaps, even a tad jealous. I'm proud of her success yet feel bad about my lack of success. It's not personal. It's just not fair.

    **c.** Inspired! This just encourages me to realize the success she's made of her life is a testament to the power of hard work, courage, willingness, and persistence. It's time to get my butt in gear! No more excuses!

**8.** If I feel anxiety about my finances, I will:

    **a.** Stop spending. Period. I will go without, even if it means depriving myself for a little while. I don't really need new things, anyway. I have all that I need and then some.

    **b.** If I really want something, I will figure out how to get it—even if it means putting it on credit or borrowing the money. I somehow always pull it off. Things just always work out for me. Someway!

c. Do a serious assessment of the situation to see if my anxiety is justified. If necessary, I will downsize and/or look for a higher-paying job. I have to face the music head-on and seek solutions to make sure my needs are always met. I am financially independent.

9. I met my (now) spouse when I was quite young. Neither of us brought much into the marriage financially, but over the years he/she has worked very hard to give us a good life, while I've been home raising the children. Recently, I noticed many of our assets are in his/her name only. I:

a. Trust that (s)he knows what (s)he's doing. I have never managed a lot of money before; (s)he probably knows best. Besides, (s)he always gives me a weekly allowance to purchase groceries and household needs. I don't go without.

b. Secretly tell my family and friends how pissed I am. They all suggest I confront him/her and demand my name be added to everything . . . but I'm afraid. Truth be told, if we break up, half of everything is mine anyway.

c. Gather as much information as possible and calmly talk to him/her about it. I believe we should each have our own credit scores and bank account, although all of our purchases over the years should clearly be in both of our names. If (s)he objects, I will follow through with outside financial and/or legal advice.

10. If a conversation with someone leaves me feeling upset or confused, I will:

a. Most likely blame myself. It's not worth saying anything. I'll get over it eventually and let bygones be bygones. Why ruffle any feathers? I'm an accepting person.

**b.** Stew for a while and then e-mail or text him or her to explain how frustrated I feel. He/she needs to take personal inventory of him/herself and his/her actions. If I don't share my feelings, how will people know they've hurt me?

**c.** I will look at why this person could upset me so much and try to find the lesson in it. Sometimes a little time and space puts things into perspective. If absolutely necessary for the sake of *saving* the relationship, I will e-mail or call so we can meet and address my feelings in a calm way.

11. My older kids rarely keep their rooms clean. I:

**a.** Argue with them to clean up but will probably end up cleaning them myself. I will not have messy rooms in my home, and it's easier to clean them myself than keep fighting with my kids.

**b.** Know where they get it from—I think my bedroom may be messier than theirs are.

**c.** Shut their bedroom doors. Unless something is growing mold, it's not my problem. I don't have to sleep in it. And my room is stunning. They'll learn eventually.

12. When I spend time with my in-laws, I usually leave feeling:

**a.** Exhausted. I try to help, whether it's preparing dinner, assisting in the cleanup, babysitting the kids, listening to problems and challenges, etc. I want my in-laws to see me as a good addition to the family.

**b.** Upset. I know they don't like me. I know they wish my spouse had married someone else. No matter what I say or do, I never feel good enough. I wish I didn't have to visit them.

   **c.** Fine. I visit when I can, leave when I want to, and enjoy
   our time together. And if I don't get along with certain
   in-laws, I simply don't visit. My partner certainly can,
   but I don't have to. I live and let live.

13. I've been married for over six years, and things have be-
    come very boring and routine. It's been years since we've
    had any kind of passion. I:

   **a.** Made a vow for better or worse. Love is a commitment
   not a feeling. Besides, I'm so tired at the end of the day,
   I can't imagine having to add "crazy sex" to my to-do
   list.

   **b.** Spend time flirting with old lovers and new admirers
   on Facebook. If my partner won't take care of me, I will.
   I'm not sure if I see this relationship lasting forever. I'm
   married not buried.

   **c.** Refocus my energy on me. It takes two to tango, and I'm
   not feeling as sensual or romantic as I used to, either. I'm
   certain he/she must be as lonely as I am. I'm sure that
   once I get my mojo back, my relationship will have some
   renewed energy. If I need to, I will schedule an appointment with a coach or therapist to talk about it.

14. A friend calls to borrow money. She's desperate. She's bor-
    rowed from me in the past and never paid me back. I:

   **a.** Give her the money. How can I say no, especially if I
   can afford it? I feel sorry for her. I know she is having a
   rough time. I just can't tell anyone I'm doing this again.

   **b.** Avoid her calls and don't answer the door when she
   comes by. I'm not the bank. I can't deal with this. She is
   going to have to grow up and figure her life out.

   **c.** Try to empower her to take control of her situation, letting her know that I believe in her ability to sort this out.
   Without drama or guilt, I offer to help her write a great

résumé or set up a meeting with a financial planner or bank officer, but I won't give her any more money.

15. If I'm facing a huge loss, I will:

   a. Keep going. It is what it is. Life goes on. Time heals all things. I try not to think about it (although my brain is always worrying).

   b. Cocoon myself. Perhaps pour myself a stiff drink, pop a pill, or eat a bowl of ice cream and pull the blankets over my head. Hopefully, this too shall pass . . . and soon.

   c. Reach out to friends, talk it out with a therapist or coach, and spend time writing in a journal. Sharing is caring. Community builds immunity. Dealing with my pain and suffering is the best way to heal it. It's hard to see it in the moment, but there are always lessons in loss.

16. I wake up feeling under the weather. Something isn't quite right. I:

   a. Try not to give any power to it. I have a busy day and there's no time to be sick. I pop a painkiller and get on with it. I'd have to be dying before I took time off work.

   b. Call my doctor to see if I can get an appointment immediately. If not, I'll go to the walk-in clinic. Better to deal with it before it turns into something bigger. I've had too many health setbacks in the past.

   c. Listen to my body. If intervention is needed, I'll try a naturopathic approach before taking anything pharmaceutical. I don't overdramatize, but I don't ignore my body's cries for attention.

17. I'm out on a first date with someone I'm extremely attracted to. The entire evening has gone as close to perfectly as possible. At the end of the date, he/she wants to "get a room." I:

a. Say no, although inside I'm secretly tickled pink! Anyone who sleeps with someone on the first date is giving the message (s)he's easy. If I plan on getting married, I'd better act like marriage material.

b. Don't hesitate! Love, love, love is all you need! Our attraction is undeniable, and I know (s)he is clearly into me! I'll be his/her sexiest lover ever, keeping my fingers crossed (s)he'll call me tomorrow.

c. Check with my internal radar. If I really want to and my gut instinct says yes, I will (as long as one of us has a condom for protection). But there's a much greater chance I'll leave him/her with the juiciest kiss and make plans for a second date.

18. When describing my sex drive/sex life, I feel:

a. Disconnected. Life is so busy; there is so much to take care of. I would love to get my sex drive back, but right now it's just not a priority.

b. Powerful. I love sex and I know the power I wield when it comes to sex. I admit I sometimes have sex just to feel better about myself.

c. Healthy and vibrant. Pleasuring myself or sharing an intimate connection with someone I care about is an important aspect of my life.

19. If someone were to describe my appearance, I think they'd see me as:

a. Simple, modest, understated, and perhaps even a little older than my chronological age. (At least that's how I feel sometimes.)

b. Someone who stands out and makes a statement. I like to be unique and to express myself through my appearance. I always seem to get attention.

    **c.** Attractive, confident, classy, and subtly sexy but never sleazy. Others often comment on how great I look.

**20.** When it comes to heterosexual, same-sex friendships, I:

    **a.** Would love to have more friends and hang out more often, but life is just too busy. It's not that I don't want to make time for friends; I just don't know where to fit it into my busy schedule.

    **b.** Prefer to have platonic friends of the *opposite* sex. I find same-sex friendships too hard. There is always jealousy or competition or something "weird." I just don't like it. Opposite-sex friendships are easier.

    **c.** Love my same-sex friends! I can't imagine my life without them. At least once a month, we get together whether to take a walk, to play sports, or to go for lunch, dinner, or a drink.

Total up all your (a) answers - _____

Total up all your (b) answers - _____

Total up all your (c) answers - _____

You may notice you have answers in all three categories (a, b, and c); each represents one of the Dominant Emotional Archetypes or an Emotional Age. Before reading each of their descriptions, pay attention to the different aspects of life that each question represented: your relationships personally, professionally, with your self, and within the community.

Remember, your Dominant Emotional Archetype has nothing to do with Chronological Age or whether you are actually a parent. For example, you could be twenty-five years old, childless, and single (even still living at home) and still completely embody the Parent Archetype—selfless, giving, overextended. On the other hand, you could be sixty years old, married with three children and ten grandchildren, and be behaving as the Child Archetype—dramatic, difficult, and overly emotional.

We all have *all three archetypes* within us, although for most of us one will be more dominant in specific areas of our lives. For example, you may be the Parent with your children or boss, the Child with your money or significant other, but the Adult with your friends or coworkers. The purpose of the quiz is to help you understand where your tendencies are guiding you so that you can figure out where to begin looking for a better, empowered balance.

Let's get back to your answers . . .

**IF YOU HAD MOSTLY (A) ANSWERS, YOUR DOMINANT EMOTIONAL ARCHETYPE IS THE PARENT (MOTHER OR FATHER ENERGY).** Your survival story is that your life is in the service of others. In fact, you spend so much time and energy providing for everyone that you have little energy left to take care of yourself. You function as if your needs and feelings don't matter—that somehow being selfless is so important that it comes before self-care. You've been taught to worry about others to the point you forget about yourself. You're not quite sure how things got so challenging, but it feels like you've always been taking care of someone—even if you don't have children of your own. Too busy being busy . . . something has to change. You will always be a giver, but you need to remember to give more to yourself so you don't burn out.

**IF YOU HAD MOSTLY (B) ANSWERS, YOUR DOMINANT EMOTIONAL ARCHETYPE IS THE CHILD (DAUGHTER OR SON ENERGY).** Games, games, and more games! Your survival story is that life is a constant power struggle filled with drama and dysfunction. But you are so tired of being insecure, competitive, and angry. You are a good person at heart, but the little voice in your head rarely turns off, constantly comparing yourself to others, which makes you often appear spoiled, sucky, or selfish. Unless you learn to grow up, life isn't going to get better! The good news is that once you learn how to expand your emotions rather than contract into them, you will find freedom.

**IF YOU HAD MOSTLY (C) ANSWERS, YOUR DOMINANT EMOTIONAL ARCHETYPE IS THE ADULT (WOMAN OR MAN ENERGY).** Congratulations! You've totally got your groove on! You know who you are and where you're going! You've done the work; rewritten the script, ignited your hidden strengths and rerouted misdirected fear into living your fullest. You are authentic, assertive, empowered, independent, strong, determined, loving, accepting, and open-minded; your reality is reflecting to you great health, wealth, love, relationships, and purpose! You feel expansive, safe, and excited about your future! You know how much you matter.

*NOTE: If your life is* not *reflecting back to you great health, wealth, love, relationships, and purpose, take the quiz again and get out of denial (didn't even notice I am lost). You must tell yourself the truth!*

Now that you understand more about Emotional Age, let's have a look at the Empowerment Spectrum, most specifically our Three Dominant Archetypes!

# CHAPTER TWO

# Three Dominant Archetypes

## "FEEL"

> It's not what you look at that matters,
> it's what you see.
>
> HENRY DAVID THOREAU

As I briefly mentioned already, the Empowerment Spectrum is the tool I created to help determine Emotional Age. It is composed of two primary concepts. The first is that we each embody Three Dominant Archetypes—the Parent, the Child, and the Adult. And the second is that we each have a style we use to engage with all those with whom we have a relationship. I call this the Communication Scale. It runs up through the center of the Empowerment Spectrum.

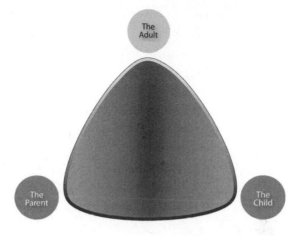

We will discuss the Communication Scale in the next chapter. In this chapter, let's focus on the Three Dominant Archetypes . . .

## What Are Archetypes?

Archetypes are not new; they have been around for centuries. Whether ancient Greek or Roman gods or goddesses representing power or weakness, mischief or love, or the saints and angels who represent divinity and strength, archetypes are timeless personas that help create shortcuts for our minds.

Archetypes make it possible to examine beliefs, attitudes, emotions, and behaviors in ways that go far beyond conventional, qualitative ways. With a simple image we conjure up a multitude of qualities or characteristics. Maybe that is the reason why we don't dream about words and sentences but rather about plots with characters that may appear somewhat surreal or even mythical. Stories, symbols, and metaphors make it easier for our brains to make sense of things. They help us achieve order and consistency.

For example, take a moment and allow your mind to think about Aphrodite or Hercules. Don't you instantly picture a beautiful, fit woman wearing a white toga and exuding love, pleasure, and fertility; and a gorgeous, muscular, sort of dopey man wearing a white tunic and doing good deeds with a god-like strength?

Now how about imagining a few real-life archetypes such as the Bad Boy or the Seductress? We're probably all picturing the same kind of person, and we might even have somebody specific in mind!

The spiritual teacher Caroline Myss, writes in her book *Archetypes*:

> I have long believed that it is impossible for us to know who we truly are unless we understand archetypes and, more specifically, our own personal archetypes, because archetypes are the psychic lenses through which we view ourselves and the world around us. As a society we have been on a quest to understand how we function psychologically, what makes us the way we are, and what makes us heal. These questions have awakened a need in us to not only be aware that archetypes influence us but how they express themselves in our individual lives. Archetypes are the new language of power."

## Why "Three" Archetypes?

The idea of humans having *three* aspects to our personality is not new. Sigmund Freud described the triad in this way:

1. The "superego," which plays the critical and moralizing role.
2. The "id," which is the set of uncoordinated instinctual trends (pure instincts).
3. The "ego," which is the organized, realistic part that mediates between the desires of the id and the superego.

Even though many of Freud's beliefs have come to be viewed in some recent psychology books as, perhaps, too sexually based, I see similarities between the id and the Child Archetype, the superego and the Parent Archetype, and the ego as the Adult Archetype—the healthy balance between id and superego.

Then there was the brilliant psychologist Carl Jung. Although his theories were different from Freud's, Jung also suggested that the psyche was composed of *three* components:

1. The "collective unconscious" is made up of archetypes and emotional symbols that are common to all individuals, i.e., religions, dreams, fairy tales, and literature from all over the world have universal meaning and understanding.
2. The "personal unconscious" or "the shadow" holds sheltered private experiences, feelings, and urges that have been actively repressed due to threatening behavior. Jung acknowledged Freud's theory that the unconscious is a storehouse for suppressed experiences from an individual's memories.
3. The "ego," also known as the Self, which is the last element in the psyche, is responsible for our feelings of identity. Jung acknowledged Freud's theory that the ego develops around age four.

The Canadian psychologist Eric Berne, founder of Transactional Analysis, first introduced the concept of the Adult,
Parent, and Child as ego states in the 1970s. He came to the
conclusion that people shift from one "ego state" to another.
Although his concepts vary greatly from the Three Dominant
Archetypes in this book, in his own work with patients he noticed that "at any given moment each individual in a social ag-
gregation will exhibit a Parental, Adult or Child ego state . . .
and individuals can shift with varying degrees of readiness
from one state to another."

Even in Christianity, we see the Father, the Son, and the
Holy Spirit as a *trinity*—collectively creating what many refer
to as "God."

Let's look now in greater detail at the Three Dominant
Archetypes of the Empowerment Spectrum.

Remember, each archetype—the Parent, the Child, and
the Adult—teaches us something or brings something of value
into our lives! We are meant to have aspects of each of these
archetypes as part of our personal archetype. The secret, you
will learn, is balancing, embodying, and expanding the lower
two—the Parent and the Child Archetypes—so that we may
transcend into the fully conscious, empowered Adult.

The descriptions of the archetypes are a touch tongue-in-
cheek, designed to make you smile while you're self-reflecting.
They will help you recognize the dominant qualities each archetype naturally embodies that, if integrated, can help you
become an authentic, whole, empowered Adult. It isn't about
rejecting or shaming any of them; it is so you can pay attention
to where they've allowed their "natural gifts" to contract into
the smallness of their fears rather than expanding into their
greatness!

Once you can acknowledge and then accept these disempowered aspects of yourself that are causing you to sabotage yourself (even unconsciously), you can start to take back control by being mindful in your communication, rising in your level of empowerment!

## THE PARENT ARCHETYPE

What immediately comes to mind when you think of Mother? Perhaps words like *giving, caring, nurturing, supportive,* and *integrity.* Father signifies *protection, strength, dependability, service,* and *reliable.*

Unfortunately, *bliss, fun, joy,* and *pleasure* are not words the Parent Archetype often identifies with. Perhaps *responsibility, stress, rescuing,* and *exhaustion* are more in the Parent's comfort zone.

Although the Parent Archetype is the most selfless of all the archetypes, selflessness doesn't always equate with happiest or most harmonious. Sometimes overgiving creates resentment and a lack of appreciation. Self-abnegating to a fault, the Parent Archetype puts everyone else first—children (if there are any), work, partner, parents, pets, friends, neighbors, community, and commitments—which means the Parent Archetype isn't always the most fun to hang out with. They're so busy taking care of others that they forget to take care of themselves. Who has the time?

The simplest way to explain the Parent Archetype is "chronic neglect of Self."

The Parent Archetype is an outcome-oriented person rather than a process-oriented person, meaning it is not the journey that counts, it's about getting the job done as efficiently and effectively as possible. *And there is always a job to do!* Most likely, they learned to be caretakers at a young age. They learned that taking care of others was the way to feel valued; putting out fires was something they did well. People counted on them, and that gave them a sense of purpose, importance, and value.

These individuals have a difficult time honoring their own feelings, needs, or desires. They feel bad about taking care of themselves when there are so many others who need their help. The needs of others are always more important than their own. Doing what is right is always more important than doing what is right for them.

Both men and women who resonate in the Parent Archetype feel that "giving" is the most important value to possess. What most don't realize is that "giving *up*" oneself is different from "giving *of*" oneself. "Giving *up*" leaves a person drained and, eventually, empty. "Giving *of*" oneself allows us to share our gifts and talents with the world, while at the same time being refilled. Individuals who resonate in the Parent Archetype, unfortunately, give up themselves.

Self–care and self–love are concepts the Parent Archetype wants to embrace. It's possible that they pass these values along to the people for whom they are caring; they just have no idea how to fit into their busy schedules attention directed toward themselves.

If the Parent Archetype is motivated to eat well and exercise, it is highly likely they do it for the purpose of living longer and staying strong and healthy so they can take care of their loved ones. It certainly isn't to fit into a new sexy black dress or to show their abs off at the gym! In fact, you'll rarely find the Parent Archetype showing off anything.

Letting loose and letting their hair down can be challenging for the Parent Archetype. Now don't get me wrong—the Parent Archetype wants to have fun and is often organizing the party, but they themselves aren't partying! They're sitting on the sidelines, scanning the crowd to make sure that everyone is having fun, or they're cooking the food and doing the dishes. It's okay! They're good at it! And they know it. Besides, the Parent Archetype doesn't want anyone to see them sweat! They avoid letting others see their wounds, insecurities, and flaws. In their mind, they have to be strong, but they don't realize that it is their selflessness that is robbing everyone—themselves and their lover—of a deeply intimate, honest, vulnerable, and connected relationship.

The underlying struggle with many people who personify this archetype is in part due to the Imposter Syndrome. I'm certain I carried it in most aspects of my life, including my intimate relationships: I rarely felt worthy, so I convinced myself I had to prove I was lovable or, at the very least, good enough. This meant being a performer in the bedroom, a gourmet chef in the kitchen, a martyr with my children, and the "hostess with the mostess" to my in-laws. I was the Stepford Wife! I was the Perfectionist! I was the Martyr! In fact, I was most of the Parent Emotional Sub-Archetypes from the Wallflower to the Mad Scientist! (You'll read about these in the next section.) Being in love exhausted rather than empowered me.

Don't get me wrong: the Parent Archetype wants to be more playful. They want to feel acceptance, joy, and peace. They don't want to be so heavy and stressed out. They want to laugh more and be lighthearted. But they can't because life isn't about their needs, wants, and feelings. The Parent is saving the world—and most likely, saving you, as well. This is serious work. Life is serious work.

This isn't a put-down, but if *happiness is the secret sauce to staying in love* and the Parent Archetype won't protect their own happiness, it's challenging to be in an intimate, close, fulfilling relationship with them.

## THE PARENT SUB-ARCHETYPES

People who embody the Parent Archetypes fall into one (or more) of the following Parent Emotional Sub-Archetypes:

1. The Wallflower
2. The Martyr
3. The Rescuer
4. The Worrywart
5. The Chubby Bubby
6. The Micromanager
7. The Busy Bee
8. The Puritan
9. The Perfectionist
10. The Ruler
11. The Mad Scientist

Outlined on the following pages are short descriptions of all the Parent Emotional Sub-Archetypes. As you read through, pay attention to where you relate to some of the same primary power issues or personal challenges of the different archetypes, including their underlying struggles with empowerment, but don't take it all too seriously. You may also notice your family members or friends in some of these Emotional Sub-Archetypes.

Recognizing yourself in some of the following Emotional Sub-Archetypes will help you to see how you are showing up in the world. You are the "cause," and reality is the "effect."

You may never discover why you chose your particular Emotional Sub-Archetype, and the truth is, it doesn't matter why. Each archetype teaches us something. Once you know better, you can do better!

The purpose of reading through all of these Emotional

Sub-Archetypes is to help you identify the characteristics or qualities that are shaping how you experience the world.

### The Wallflower

See that faded silhouette amid the shadows in the background? That's the Wallflower. Without reluctance, individuals who exemplify this archetype commit themselves to a seat in the audience, while allowing others the full attention onstage. Although they have the potential to be brilliant showstoppers themselves, Wallflowers tend to tuck away their own shiny traits as if treasures for safekeeping.

Phenomenal listeners, Wallflowers are silent supporters who are always careful not to overshadow others. They wouldn't want to steal anyone's thunder. They are the ever-willing volunteers standing behind the camera of that group photo or quietly cleaning up the messes that others make, never expecting so much as a pat on the back. Most of us don't even realize Wallflowers are there or that they've done so much work. Blending in is their strategy.

They are people watchers. Since they always stand back, they capture a broad view of life as it is happening and seem to remember everything, with no details spared. They are actually some of the best at reminiscing and telling stories . . . if you can get them talking!

When it comes to understanding human interactions, Wallflowers are unsure and awkward. Truth be told, *awkward* is a word they themselves may use when describing how they feel trying to network or socialize at public events. Some may call them shy or introverted, but in reality, they are uncomfortable in a group setting. A good percentage of them are actually hoping that you won't even look at them, let alone talk to them. As a result, they tend to stay isolated. Wallflowers are extremely passive; and wish they could join in and make friends more easily.

### The Martyr

Martyrs are servile, compliant, and submissive. They have been taught to be the wind beneath everyone else's wings. As young people, they developed an unbelievably keen sense of knowing what others want and can usually deliver, even when it's for another person's cravings or desires (especially those that shouldn't be indulged). Martyrs might know that it's not a good idea to enable our vices, but they feel too guilty to say no.

Martyrs are incredibly supportive and loyal, sometimes to a fault. They'll stay in relationships, situations, and jobs that demean and discourage them just because it's the right thing to do. Martyrs won't rock the boat. They never want anyone to be sad, angry, hurt, or hungry. Besides, there's nothing a good meal can't fix. They will cook and clean and cook some more. They will give up their last dollar, their last meal, their own bed, even their dignity, if you ask for it. They just want to help. *Deep down*, Martyrs want to take better care of themselves (although they rarely dig that deep, unless gardening). They aren't satisfied with their life but feel guilty even considering this notion. They simply have no idea how to put themselves first. They've been responsible for so long, they don't know any other way. Without fail, the kids, job, partner, parents, siblings, pets, boss, coworkers, neighbors, errands, meals, laundry, cleaning, shopping, volunteering, PTA meetings, bake sales, friends, babysitting, you name it—even strangers—come before them. Always. Period.

Martyrs are exhausted at the end of the day. They swear they are going to make changes, but they simply don't know how. Martyrs are beautiful souls who want only the best for everyone; they have just forgotten what best means for them-selves. They certainly aren't going to question God or dare ask for more. Spoiled, selfish people do that. Not the Martyrs!

If they do get upset, it doesn't last long—at least not on the surface. Martyrs know to turn the other cheek and show the world what being humble, meek, and selfless looks like. Con-frontation is to be avoided at all costs. If they are upset, they'll bury it. No point in crying over spilled milk (although they'll clean that up, too).

### The Rescuer

Nursing and mending their flock of wounded sheep, Res-cuers surround themselves with people who need to be fixed or saved.

With an effortless ability to find broken people, it would seem that they are drawn to the *wounded* and the *wounded* are drawn to them. Unsure of how to connect with a person unless they can somehow help, Rescuers require you to be broken; once you are fixed, Rescuers are unsure how to maintain the relationship. Don't get me wrong: Rescuers are really good people! They welcome anyone with open arms, an open heart, and an open mind. Actually, they welcome you with an *open everything*: an open front door, an open schedule, an open wal-let, and mostly, wide-open boundaries. Come in and stay as long as you need (and this goes for absolutely any of the Emo-tional Sub-Archetypes). There is no one Rescuers won't help!

In fact, take whatever you need but only as long as you're broken. Once you're back on track, they may lose interest in you. Don't take it personally. You're no longer wounded, and there are so many others whom they can help. They must move on. In a bizarre way, it is only sad stories and broken people who tend to last as friends with these individuals. Become too strong and you may not need them . . . and that is a no-no! Being needed is their number one priority.

Rescuers' modus operandi is to find an entryway into an old wound. By awakening the inner victim and by encouraging us to give past pains and suffering excessive attention, Rescuers are able to get to work. They seem to thrive talking and focusing on other people's problems. Maybe doing so makes them feel better about themselves. Focusing on others certainly allows them not to think about their own needs or feelings.

Although they are as reliable as the rising sun, sometimes their help may not seem like help at all, but rather an imposition. If ever someone becomes frustrated with their involvement, Rescuers are left to wonder what they did that was so terribly wrong . . . *After all, they were just trying to help!*

Readily available to a fault, Rescuers want nothing more than to help you succeed. The trouble is, this Parent Archetype helps and helps until you feel suffocated. Can we say "codependent"?

*Codependent* is a term first used by Melody Beattie, in her book *Codependent No More*, to describe a person who enables alcoholics and drug addicts to stay dependent on their vice of choice. By focusing on someone with substance abuse issues, a codependent person makes the addict his or her *own* "addiction." If the addict is good, the codependent is good. If the addict has fallen off the wagon, it becomes the codependent person's life purpose to save him or her again. *This is how the Rescuers live their lives, as well.*

Taking responsibility for that which is not theirs, this archetype is most likely to react to and speak as though another's successes, and even more so another's *failures*, are all their own. They are simply too involved, so they personalize everything.

They can't help but overstep boundaries, although rest assured, their intentions are centered solely on the well-being and betterment of others. If only they could expand their Emotional Edges, they could become incredible Light Protectors! (We'll talk more about this "career strategy" in Chapter Eight.)

### The Worrywart

Can't sleep at night, racing thoughts always consuming you, worried about the "what–ifs"? Maybe you are a Worrywart!

None of us is exempt from a worry-free life, but for Worrywarts, they cannot seem to operate without worrying about everything. These nervous wrecks get stuck in their relentless ruminations, overwhelmed, navigating their lives with the future's possible catastrophes constantly on their minds.

Not to mention, guard your bubbles closely, because when Worrywarts are around, they unknowingly may burst them, as well: "I'm worried it won't work" is their most common sentiment.

According to Worrywarts, most things don't work. It's just the unavoidable pitfall of life. No matter the circumstances, no matter how certain you are about your plans, they discourage any type of risky business—which could even include traveling or going on adventures. (Car accidents often happen within five miles of home, you know! You need to be safe!)

Regardless of how incredible and certain you feel in your choices, you can be sure that Worrywarts will find a reason to tell you that it's not a good idea. In their minds, they're just trying to save you the trouble of hurting yourself. They're worried about you!

The challenge with Worrywarts is they've gotten into the habit of always finding something to worry about so there's little room left over to have fun; their brains are consumed with thinking about the potential problems and pitfalls that may hurt their loved ones.

If you ask them why they worry so much, you see that all this anxiety is not an act: they truly believe they are simply doing their due diligence, sometimes even worrying to the point of having anxiety attacks. And the fact that you aren't worrying stresses them out even more!

Unfortunately, acting preemptively is how they remain perpetually stuck in a state of stress and, at times, unruly panic. Ten steps ahead, they've already begun planning an exit strategy before an opportunity has even had a chance to take off.

Living in varying degrees of fear, a lot of which is irrational, Worrywarts don't trust their ability to handle whatever life has in store for them, especially since they've determined that life is an unsafe place to be. Sadly, this archetype is so weary and burdened that those who are Worrywarts often become a burden to their loved ones, even though all they want is to prevent others' pain. Eventually, their downright neuroticism—refusing to let go and move forward—begins to affect everyone they touch. It's exhausting hanging out with Worrywarts. God bless them!

### The Chubby Bubby

One may believe that excess body weight is merely the manifestation of overeating, but for the Chubby Bubbies the extra fat represents a belief system that close to 50 percent of the population seems to have adopted.

In an honest moment, the Chubby Bubbies would profess that, although looking thin appears to be the goal, "being thin" feels too vulnerable. This archetype has a certain sense of strength that they believe is rarely witnessed in thin, overly emotional people—people who feel too much!

So Chubby Bubbies have figured out a brilliant way to create an emotional buffer or filter, keeping other people's emotions and drama at "arm *and belly* length." Their extra size literally shelters them from feeling the weight of the world. Yet, in an honest moment, they would admit they do take on the weight of the world—and have for most of their lives. Bottom line, being thin is too stressful, unsafe, and overwhelming, and yet, being thin is all they dream about becoming.

Chubby Bubbies prefer to call themselves "Emotional Eaters" when, in fact, this archetype's struggle has less to do with food and more to do with cortisol—the body's stress hormone. "Stress" is their middle name, and although the Chubby Bubbies have learned how to numb most of it by not feeling, they can't fool their metabolisms.

With their bodies constantly releasing adrenaline (the precursor to cortisol, which is the pillar of aging and obesity), the Chubby Bubbies' adrenal glands are exhausted and depleted. So no matter how many diets they go on or how many miles they walk, the Chubby Bubbies remain chubby. Besides, what does it hurt? The extra body fat helps them feel larger, stronger, more stable, and unshakable. Not to mention, it helps bring less attention to them, even making them less threatening and more likable. *"Yes, my being fat"* they believe, *"makes other people feel better about themselves."* So, in part, this is a typical Parent Archetype: better that you feel good about yourself when you're around them than that they feel good about themselves.

In their heart of hearts, though, the Chubby Bubbies hate the excess weight more than anyone, but they just can't seem to lose it, even if they exercise daily and live on a diet! And most Chubby Bubbies do live on diets.

Most days, they look into the mirror or stand on the scale, self-punishing and self-loathing. No one could be meaner to the Chubby Bubbies than the Chubby Bubbies. You can't imagine the way they talk to themselves! The internal battle is debilitating: lose weight and feel too much (and possibly shine too brightly)? Or stay fat, safe, and sheltered but continue the self-loathing?

If they are in a relationship, it's often viewed as one that's safe, stable, and secure, more of a friend than a lover. The Chubby Bubbies try desperately to convince everyone, even themselves, that they aren't missing out on anything! These individuals wish they felt sexier but, in truth, sexy stuff embarrasses them. Sexy lingerie, sex toys, or sexy conversation is not something they are willing to try on themselves. It's all very uncomfortable. And it doesn't matter how many other sexy people they see who carry extra weight—women or men who "walk it, talk it, and still have a tantalizing love life"—Chubby Bubbies are convinced they are different. Certain that if they could just lose weight, they'd be comfortable showing their sexuality; instead, they wear each of their unwanted pounds like shackles that chain them to their protection.

The Chubby Bubbies try to stay safe—staying in the comfort zone rather than risking it by trying to be too sexy. Offering fantastic companionship but not daring to try for romantic fulfillment.

### The Micromanager

Feeling like the back of your neck is getting a little hot and humid? That's because the Micromanager is breathing down it! This archetype makes sure to oversee everything at an uncomfortably close distance.

The Micromanagers sweat the small stuff and want you to

sweat it with them! Relentless harassing, harping, hounding, and badgering, this archetype sounds more like a broken record than an empowered motivator! Some may even call them a nag!

What Micromanagers don't seem to recognize is that the more they pester, the more they're disrespected. Unsure of how to speak to others in a way that gets anyone's needs met, those falling within this archetype are unable to pick their battles wisely. Instead, Micromanagers get caught up in the details, nitpicking and complaining about everything and anything that crosses their mind.

Underestimating other people's competence is their specialty; so is overestimating their own ability to deal with pressure, stress, and—let's be honest—people in general. They aren't great team players, nor are they successful as team leaders. They just can't seem to let go of the reins, on even the tiniest details. Can you say "Control freak"?

Under the circumstances of having to manage others, such as running a household or coordinating a business team, the Micromanagers have a strong need to control the entire process at large. They will reluctantly hand over responsibilities only when they have no other choice. But you can be sure that if Micromanagers must assign tasks to others, it is not without first going completely overboard in providing *majorly* detailed instructions.

With the best of intentions, Micromanagers desperately fear that others will mess up, and so they are simply trying to provide as much information as possible, but with so many expectations and instructions it has the opposite effect: most people feel as though they've gone into a state of data overload with this detail-oriented, can't-let-go-of-the-reins, person.

In fact, Micromanagers often end up getting worse work

from people because of the overexplaining. In the end, the only people who last with Micromanagers are those with no independent creativity because everybody else gets so frustrated with not having a voice, they walk away.

The Micromanagers are also unbelievably preoccupied with how others' actions will reflect back on them. Known for driving people batty with endless update requests, we often spend most of our time reporting back to and checking in with them rather than actually progressing at an acceptable pace.

When things aren't going according to plan, they are some of the most difficult people to be around since they tend to be ticking time bombs: hyper-reactive, with a low threshold for stress, the Micromanagers inevitably make mountains out of molehills. When things go wrong, you can count on Micromanagers to panic rather than look for solutions. They are so consumed with the details, they simply can't see the bigger picture. Holding on tightly, they believe that gripping, forcing, and overmanaging others will eventually pay off. But it never does.

### The Busy Bee

The Busy Bees never stop! There is always something important to do! In fact, if you have to get something done, just give it to a Busy Bee. No matter how much is on their plate, they are happy and willing to take on more!

With not a minute to waste, the Busy Bees' schedules are filled from morning to night; there's just so much to get done, and although they may pencil in downtime, they're only kidding themselves. Anyone who knows a Busy Bee knows they can't relax. They may intend to sit down with a cup of hot tea but will end up spotting the dust on the light fixture that hangs above their table. It's only after they've dusted *every* light fixture in the house that they'll take a sip of their now-cold tea. Oh well, that's just the way the Busy Bees buzz!

You can have the best time with this archetype, if you *aren't* looking for an intimate connection or deep, emotional conversations; Busy Bees are always more than willing to stay busy and get involved in every project (not to mention, some Busy Bees are quite adventurous).

*"I'm in"* are two words most favored by the Busy Bees— and for many friends, this is the ultimate companion! But unfortunately, if you want to share a deeper relationship with these individuals, you may be left feeling disappointed, even a little stung with their inability to make you—or your feelings—a priority. They just have too much on the go! "It's not personal," they'll assure you—they are just so in demand with all of their responsibilities and commitments!

Too busy being busy, this archetype is often so in denial of their inability to feel their own feelings, take care of their own emotional baggage, or face the music of their past, let alone get into heavy conversation about your feelings, baggage, or past. Sadly, they don't have the self-awareness to realize that they're sacrificing deep personal relationships in favor of superficial time fillers because they're afraid of "feeling." Instead, they'd rather just buzz along, "collecting pollen," so to speak, staying out of trouble and making sweet honey! Besides, if you bug them too much, they'll just sting you and fly off!

On top of it all, the Busy Bees often mistake being productive with being busy. Instead of working on their business plan, you'll find them decorating the kitchen or playing a game of golf. Instead of finishing the project that has the looming deadline, they'll choose to meet a friend for lunch or grab some groceries. Instead of getting up and heading straight to the gym for their workout, they'll open up their computer and get lost in Facebook (or something else just as trivial). They just can't say no: "Jack of all trades, master of none!"

The Busy Bees mean no harm, but their inability to slow down and truly connect hinders their love relationships. They have too much on their agenda for that! Don't expect to peg them down long enough to have that serious, intimate talk! Let's keep the train moving!

Unaware that they continuously choose things, people, or activities that give them a temporary "high"—immediate satisfaction—over self-reflecting and properly prioritizing, the Busy Bees may not realize how often they replace high-priority actions with less-important distractions. All of which, interferes with their ability to fulfill their own life's purpose, as well.

### The Puritan

"Cleanliness is next to godliness," and Puritans are squeaky clean! These God-fearing, volunteering, good-hearted, right fighters have lived their whole lives dutifully climbing the stairway to heaven, and they aren't going to stop now. Propriety, purity, and etiquette (in other words, "good manners") drive this archetype!

Puritans have righteousness running through their veins and will do just about anything to be of service to their family and community. This is different from *self*-righteousness and different from Rescuers' agendas: the Puritans really want to be pure . . . and want you to be, as well! It's the "right" way! It's the only way to the pearly gates!

The Puritans feel that they have been called to lead a life of devout altruism and can often be found selflessly offering their time and efforts to those in need. Living their lives as wholesomely as possible, these good and moral people are inspired by the virtues of their Holy Book, which, at times, can make them come across as a little stuffy and old-fashioned.

It is important to note that to Puritans, the definition of *inappropriate* is more uncompromising than most people's definition. Puritans maintain a humble and modest appearance; clothing is simply the means by which we cover our nakedness, which means covering up is crucial to their image. But you may not actually notice them; these lovely people have a presence that could easily go unseen, since they are highly conscientious about making certain not to draw too much attention to themselves. They keep it clean, always!

The Puritans are on a mission to save, sacrifice, care for, and minister to those in need. The sad part is how misjudged they are by most of society. Their biggest mistake is simply in their delivery rather than in their intentions. While Puritans mean well, they can leave others feeling judged because of how strongly they hold on to their own beliefs. This can become isolating for both them and those they love most.

The hardest aspect for many of the partners (married or monogamous) of Puritans is how reserved they are sexually. "Why does sex matter so much?" Puritans wonder. "Why is this world so consumed with sex, sex, sex? There are so many more important things to think about and take care of." And so it is for the life of the Puritans.

### The Perfectionist
A+ is the only grade the Perfectionists are willing to accept. Anything less won't do, which leaves them continuously striving and trying, feeling overwhelmed and overcommitted. Unable to ask for help or to show their flaws, Perfectionists give off the impression that they do it all with ease. Looking perfect, as you can imagine, matters most, so showing others

that they are struggling would not be acceptable. *"Never let 'em see you sweat"* is their mantra. *"There's nothing I can't do!"*

The sad part is that success is rarely satisfying for Perfectionists because they are already onto the next project. Not to mention, when they look back at their own accomplishments, deep down, they feel they could always have done better, or maybe, said differently, things should always *be* better.

The real question: Are Perfectionists happy and fulfilled within themselves?

Perfectionists fall into two categories: the Self-Imposed Perfectionists and those who impose perfectionism on others.

The Self-Imposed Perfectionists are obsessed with how they do things. In their minds, they should always deliver work that is 100 percent flawless all of the time, every time. Because of this deep need to be picture perfect, they may occasionally talk themselves out of pursuing their greatest dreams, because 90 percent success would feel like a failure to them.

The Perfectionists who force their high standards on everyone in their lives can come across as dictators or tyrants. Their super-high expectations—with a right and wrong way to do everything from washing the dishes to watering the plants—create a constant pressure for the people in their lives. Not only do they make others feel inadequate for never meeting their standards (*no one* meets their standards), they form an internal message that goes something similar to this: "If I want something done right, I better do it myself!"

A fitting image to illustrate this archetype would be a woman straight out of the pages of a 1950s *Woman's Day* magazine: her home is pristine in cleanliness and decor; she is impeccably groomed; her children seem to come out of mud puddles clean; her relationships appear to be happy and highly functional; her social life is fun and lively.

Man or woman, the Perfectionists strive to be immaculate! They throw the most incredible parties and gatherings, making certain that all guests have what they need. No stomach or glass has ever gone empty on their watch.

In the meantime, Perfectionists are metaphorically lashing themselves for a job never done well enough. But you will never know. On the outside, the Perfectionists are always happy and positive. There is no room for negativity. Negativity is imperfect.

If only Perfectionists would learn that sometimes "good enough is good enough," they might actually begin to enjoy all their amazing accomplishments and expand their consciousness just enough to become Light Workers (we'll talk more about this "career strategy" in Chapter Eight).

### The Ruler

Call them Queen, King, Matriarch, or Patriarch—it's pretty much all the same; Rulers rule because they care! Rulers often find themselves in positions of authority, taking on the weight of the world. Stamina like a workhorse, if they aren't the Boss, they are the best employees in the world. Rulers are unshakable, solid, strong, and accountable; they are fearless for those in need.

Born leaders, Rulers can absolutely get the job done— although it's stressful and even oppressive to work with them. But when they take on a cause, they will make it happen . . . *because it's not about them* . . . it is about the job—the mission, the duty, the undertaking, the movement! Rulers won't drop the ball! They won't let you down! They will evoke the change you are fighting for! Rulers have important work to do and are serious about getting the job done. Intimidation and manipulation are sometimes their most effective tools at ensuring their "team" wins. Winning, rather than happiness, is what matters most.

Rulers are the "Alpha Dogs." Period. Don't cross them or you'll get bitten! Respect them . . . and they'll take care of you very well!

Strong, smart, self-righteous, and fiercely protective, this archetype knows what is right, does what is right, and will impress upon you how you should be making the right choice, as well. Criticizing, demeaning, and belittling, they believe in helping those around them become better people—and this is the strategy they know works. If only you knew . . . Under it all, Rulers have a heart of gold: tough on the outside, pure selflessness on the inside. It is all about you and for you.

Efficient, effective, and competent, Rulers want to do the best job, and if they are on your side, you can feel their intensity, dedication, and power. They dangle their love like a carrot: if you do well, they'll reward you handsomely, but if you disappoint, they will snatch their attention away until you follow the rules. There is a hierarchy in life. It's called respect, and you'd better know your place.

Rulers manifest with excessively masculine energy—even the female Rulers! These people have a hard time showing their soft, gentle, sensuous side. You won't get a lot of "warm and feely" with these people; being sensitive, they were taught, is a sign of weakness.

Nevertheless, they are dedicated to a fault; if Rulers have your back, you can be pretty certain they won't let you fall or fail. Just don't expect a warm bear hug! If only this archetype could expand their Emotional Edge, they could be amazing Light Protectors! (You'll read more about this "career strategy" in Chapter Eight.)

### The Mad Scientist

*"No great mind has ever existed without a touch of madness."*
Clearly Aristotle was familiar with the Mad Scientist!

Somehow, someway, this brilliant archetype is always in the process of working on something extremely important—world changing! The trouble with these workaholics is that what starts as exhilaration and excitement can soon become unhealthy obsession the closer they get to their "eureka." Who has time for sleep when they're on the brink of achieving absolute genius? Who has time to eat? Exercise? Plan dinner parties? Go on holidays? Have friends?

Red-eyed and unhinged, the Mad Scientists are so engulfed in their work that anything else requiring their time is actually perceived as stealing from their cause.

But the truth is, they aren't paying attention to time . . . or to you . . . or to anything other than their "purpose." They don't mean to ignore you; they can't help it. They are Mad Scientists!

Mad Scientists are fueled by an intense drive, and it appears as though the rest of their existence comes to a screeching halt whenever they take on a "cause." No matter, those who fall within this archetype willingly put their personal lives on the back burner in the name of their vision and mission.

Rarely leaving their workspace, the sun can rise and set without Mad Scientists having seen any of it. And as much as they themselves know they need to make changes to create more balance in their lives, these overachievers try to assure everyone, including themselves: "I will slow down after this next project is finished." But it never happens. There is always more genius that needs revealing.

The real trouble occurs because without a strong, healthy body—one that requires us to step away from the desk, computer, telephone, lab coat, project, etc., to exercise, play, rest, eat well, laugh, joke, and rejuvenate—Mad Scientists are putting nails in their own coffin. Yes—maybe they are saving the world, but if they don't focus more on their own health, they won't be around long enough to share their incredible gifts and talents with those they so desperately want to help!

To top it all off, *if* Mad Scientists don't focus more on their personal relationships, they may also discover that once they achieve their "eureka," they have few real friends and loved ones to celebrate it with!

Balance is most needed here! Mad Scientists would be on the brink of the Emotional Edge if they could expand their horizons just slightly! What Light Workers they could be!

No matter which Parent Archetype is being discussed, the most recognizable quality they all possess is their inability to honor their own feelings, needs, or desires. They feel bad taking care of themselves. The needs of others are always more important than their own.

If only the Parent Archetype could balance their selflessness with a little more selfishness, self-advocacy, and self-care they would feel happier, more relaxed, and empowered. Not to mention, they'd be more fun to hang out with! Besides, although others view them as noble and even saintly, they know they're flying under the radar, playing it small in their own lives. It's about time the Parent started parenting themselves better!

## THE CHILD ARCHETYPE

The Child Archetype is the complete opposite of the Parent Archetype. They need too much. Expect too much. Demand too much. Feel too much. Often extremely emotional, nothing is ever middle of the road with then.

Overwhelmed by emotion, those who embody the Child Archetype know there is more to life . . . and they want it! They just don't always know exactly what that is, what it looks like, how to receive it, or how to keep it. The fear of never knowing if their future is safe leaves them feeling frenetic and overwhelmed.

Desperate for attention and approval, under the scared, sweet, sexy, and/or tough facade are people who want acceptance, support, encouragement, and a soul mate love affair. Whether they have a partner or not, dreaming of finding "the One" is always somewhere on their agenda (even if it's hidden). They struggle to feel complete, whole, and authentic and are always looking for someone or something to fill up their missing joy.

The Child Archetype constantly searches for more, asking for more than most people can give. They create situations in which their own personal power is tested, and they constantly test the people in their lives, too. Acceptance is not something the Child Archetype does well with. Things can always be better, relationships should always be better, and other people should always be more considerate of the Child Archetype. Emotionally, they are simply immature. They can't see the bigger picture in spite of their most immediate needs. They don't know their own capabilities and are always waiting for someone to come and notice them.

Unfortunately, the Child Archetype doesn't realize they are creating their own disorders, addictions, obsessions, illnesses, syndromes, fears, phobias, and/or dysfunctions. At some point in life, this archetype has likely battled self-esteem issues resulting in alcoholism, drug use (prescription or otherwise), gambling, promiscuity, eating disorders, extreme exercising, plastic surgery, affairs, debt or bad credit, extreme loneliness, or even abusive relationships; drama follows them everywhere. But they can't see it.

In deep denial, the Child Archetype literally can't see the truth and can't be told what to do. *Ever try telling two-year-olds they can't have something?*

The power struggle can be exhausting to be around, and whether they realize it or not, others can feel their underlying hostility, no matter how friendly their facade. In the back of the mind of the Child Archetype, they're thinking: "If you hurt me, I'll hurt you."

People who resonate in the Child Archetype are rarely happy with their physiques, either. They could (and should) be leaner, more fit, and sexier. If they could change themselves, they would. Plastic surgery is always an option. Certain they would feel happier if they looked better; they always need to fix, alter, modify, and manipulate their bodies.

Now don't get me wrong, these people can bring a lot of fun and excitement to their relationships. When they are good, they are very, very good! But the extremes with this archetype can quickly turn fun into trouble and excitement into chaos. The Child can't help it. Something has happened to make them distrustful of other people. They don't want to grow up. Maybe becoming the Adult scares them because they don't want to get stuck. They need to keep all their options open.

The Child Archetype wants to make better choices, but they don't feel equipped. They don't know their own worth. Shame has wrapped around their ankles and whispered into their ears that they are no good. This is all unconscious. The Child doesn't realize how competent they actually are. They underestimate themselves constantly.

The Child Archetype exhausts everyone in the same way a high-maintenance child can deplete a parent. In time, their difficult, dramatic, and excessively needy personality destroys the relationship before it can blossom into true, everlasting love.

The *children* of the Child Archetype often treat that parent as a child. Big mistake. As immature as these people are, they don't want to be parented by anyone—especially their own children. They will fight like siblings—even rejecting their own kids—if they don't feel like they can win.

When it comes to work, the Child Archetype is usually excited beyond the moon when they first get hired, but they struggle to sustain their position. Showing up late, leaving early, the constant drama in their lives will alert even the most understanding boss that trouble is brewing!

Until those who fall within the Child Archetype actively strive to stop the drama, dysfunction, temper tantrums, mood swings, addictions, commitment issues, and/or cheating, love relationships won't work, career ideas won't blossom, and parenting children will be a disaster.

### THE CHILD SUB-ARCHETYPES

Most people who embody the Child Archetype exhibit one or more of the following Emotional Sub-Archetypes:

1. The Scared Child
2. The Addict
3. The Victim
4. The Lone Wolf
5. The Rebellious Teenager
6. The Troublemaker
7. The Drama Queen

8. The Charmer
9. The Joker
10. The Warrior
11. The Narcissist

As you read, pay attention to where you relate to or embody some of the same primary power issues or personal challenges of the different Emotional Sub-Archetypes, including their underlying struggles with empowerment, but don't take it all too seriously. Self-awareness is having the insight to recognize how you are showing up in the world—the good, the bad, and the ugly. It is not intended to shame you in any way.

As I previously mentioned, *you* are the "cause," and reality is the "effect." Your life is showing you which Emotional Sub-Archetype(s) you embody most. We can change only that which we are willing to see. Don't let *denial (didn't even notice I am lost)* prevent you from recognizing your Emotional Age—especially in stressful situations. Have some fun with this!

### The Scared Child

The Scared Child is the most fearful, helpless, and overwhelmed of all the archetypes. And although their affect may appear to be an act, it's not; these people are truly confused, unsure, and afraid. Their only survival mechanism is to attract people who will vow to take care of them for all eternity. Once they latch on, they just keep taking and taking and taking . . . until they deplete the relationship.

With little to no understanding of what healthy, Empowered Communication looks and sounds like, Scared Children have discovered a form of manipulation that works too well for them to quit. Their strategy is to need more and more and more, for as long as possible, until you put your foot down and disengage, which almost inevitably causes them to feel even more terrified, alone, and helpless.

As bad as we may feel for them, over time it is challenging to be around someone who is so insecure and needy. They constantly have their ears and eyes peeled for underlying, hurtful messages. As soon as they pick up on what they perceive to be a put-down they draw back, pull away, and find a sad corner in which to sit and sulk. Inevitably, they create the very thing they fear most: rejection.

Within the protective confines of this persona, Scared Children are able to evade responsibility, accountability, and even real-life consequences while gaining other people's sympathies. They depend on passivity and hope that you'll see them as inferior and incapable; if you view them acting like a child, you will treat them as such. You will take care of them. You will do it for them. You won't abandon them.

Scared Children know they have needs, and they know they are deserving of having those needs met. But they don't know other effective methods of making that happen—childish behavior is all they've got.

Scared Children prefer to avoid grown-up conversations or situations where they must make the decisions or be in charge. Sometimes they literally speak in baby talk or revert to tears in order to avoid responsibility in tough situations.

When forced to confront aspects of their lives that aren't working out, Scared Children think that saying "I'm not good at that" or "I don't understand" is enough to divert their responsibilities to someone else. Their insecurity is blatant. Not very empowering, especially if they have children of their own who are counting on them to be the parent.

## The Addict

Addicts struggle with the reality of their lives and have found a way to escape or temporarily numb out. The internal environment that has caused the dependency is the same across the board: *Feel bad. Indulge. Feel good. Feel bad. Indulge. Feel good. Feel bad. Indulge. And so on.*

Instead of asking themselves what feeling they're trying to escape and then implementing actions to improve their situation, they've handed over all control. The sad truth is that Addicts often believe that they never had any control to begin with.

Addicts can have one or more physiological or psychological dependencies, which often become actual addictions. The big ones are alcohol, drugs, food (resulting in eating disorders: overeating, binging, or anorexia), sex, porn, gambling, hoarding, adrenaline, and risky behavior, while shopping, religion, working, exercising, even excessive television watching or Internet surfing can blind Addicts from making changes.

Stuck in patterns, engaging in extreme behaviors to avoid "feeling certain feelings" (and remember, all addicts have specific emotions they'd do just about anything to avoid), the word *moderation* just isn't in their vocabulary.

The Addicts aren't concerned with nurturing relationships. Relationships mean "feeling"—which means caring, listening to, talking, sharing, and responding to another person's needs. Addicts are too flooded already with their own feelings to care too deeply for anyone else's feelings. Numbing it all out, in whatever way they've learned how, comes first.

Addicts don't want to hurt other people, especially their loved ones, but they can't help it. Their needs always come first. Addicts are selfish and ashamed; this is one of the issues that keeps them stuck circling the drain—never finding personal emotional empowerment. Their feelings always manage them rather than the reverse.

People who struggle with addictions depend upon others to enable them, which is why Addicts often have codependent relationships, especially with those whose Dominant Emotional Archetype is the Parent. Parent Archetypes are designed to rescue, save, and fix. Something that Addicts depend upon to exist.

What Addicts have to learn is that we must feel if we want to heal. Unfortunately, the Addict will do almost anything to stay disconnected from their pain and suffering—even if it means destroying their own life and devastating the lives of those who love them.

### The Victim

*"You will not believe what happened to me!"* is the most famous line of the Victim.

Oh yes, we will because something shockingly horrible is always happening to Victims! Their stories of abuse, neglect, injury, betrayal, and oppression are shocking and never ending. So much so that, over time, we sadly begin to question if maybe they themselves are the culprits of their own demise.

The reality is that Victims *have* been victimized. They are wounded, scared, and hurt. Their stories are true, but unfortunately, they've allowed their sad tales to define them. It's all they seem to identify with. Unable to talk about anything positive, Victims exude negativity and a "poor me" attitude. They may even feel jealous of other people's success, wondering why they themselves have had such bad luck while other people's lives are so much easier than theirs.

Without fail, it seems that Victims make a beeline for either the happiest person in a group or for Rescuers (it's bizarre how easily Victims and Rescuers always seem to find each other)! But no matter how many times you try to reach in to pull them out of their black hole, they'll grab your hand to pull you in with them.

Truth is, Victims like being in the hole, not necessarily alone, but they depend upon the attention they get while they're in it. It's cozy and comfortably familiar, even though it sucks.

The Victims don't realize they've become so accustomed to telling their trials and tribulations to anyone who will listen that they've forgotten how to have a normal conversation about normal things. Everything is about them and their problems! Everything is about their past! Everything is about who is still hurting them! They depend upon others to listen to their stories of woe and doom because they are looking for validation and camaraderie, as well as attention—something they never feel they get enough of. Misery, they have discovered, keeps them more interesting than if they were healed and whole.

Their inability to create boundaries and step outside of themselves makes it challenging for them to develop deeply personal relationships. Their *own* emotional state is all they are able to focus on. If you can talk to them about them, they're usually fine, but if it turns to anything outside of them, they will quickly close up shop and check out; it becomes too much of a drain for them.

Sadly, this means they need to find and create new woes to maintain their wounded identity (but don't ever try telling Victims that)! If you dare suggest they are even partly responsible for their constant troubles, they will see you as another victimizer in their life!

Oh . . . and if you eventually decide to stop listening, get ready: it won't matter how many wonderful things you've done for these people, you, too, will become one of the many horrendous stories they share with others.

### The Lone Wolf

Lone Wolves have unplugged almost completely from the outside world—meaning, with all of their relationships—including with their loved ones. Lone Wolves hide, retreat, and isolate, and are afraid to let anyone in. Living more like hermits, Lone Wolves have figured out how to exist with very little interaction with the outside world.

We all need to be alone at times for introspection and healing, but the Lone Wolves have given up on their pack. It's proven to be more of a hurt-filled hardship than anything else.

A lack of trust is a major issue with Lone Wolves, who feel as if the people who should have loved and protected them most have betrayed and hurt them. This archetype has a difficult time opening up and letting anyone in. "Mistrust" is their middle name.

Lone Wolves may allow one new person into their lives at a time, but should they feel hurt in any way by that person, they will cut him or her off without so much as a warning. Don't bother asking them for an explanation or offering an apology; each relationship is open and shut, and there is no room for conversation or negotiation. You'll never hear from them again. Ever. Push them too hard, and they'll lash out at you to drive you away; better they hurt you than give you a chance to hurt them.

These are incredibly loyal and devoted people, but they are also highly sensitive and easily hurt. They've experienced a rejection at a formative point in their lives, and they are struggling to protect themselves.

On top of it, without social cues and people who love us

enough to reel us in at times (or alternatively, to give us the push we need), we may all become our own worst enemy, which is what has happened to Lone Wolves: hiding away, secluded, and almost sequestered, they inevitably barricade themselves into their intense privacy, learning how to do almost everything without having to spend time with society. Friendships, shopping, even entertainment can all be done online or not at all. Real relationships—up front and personal with real people— become less and less important. Lone Wolves convince themselves that they prefer their own company; watching TV or movies, reading books, or pursuing the hobbies that interest them has offered these extremely private people the stimulation they need without the stress of commitment or accountability to others. Besides, most Lone Wolves don't consider themselves lonely. They most always have furry friends—dogs, cats, or some "mate" to call a companion.

Over time, Lone Wolves lose touch with the bigger picture; their natural ambition and sense of purpose for life become faint and distant thoughts, while their need to be disconnected from society takes precedence. Depression is all too easy to fall into, and without having any connections or obligation to show up for others, Lone Wolves can have an almost impossible time getting help.

### The Rebellious Teenager

Angry and defiant, the Rebellious Teenagers have decided the rules don't apply to them. They do what they want, dress how they want, go where they want, eat what they want, drink what they want, smoke what they want, come home when they want, and care little what anyone else thinks—regardless of who it is. They'll roll into work late (if they can keep a job), miss family functions, and play fast and loose with debts; Rebellious Teenagers are always pushing limits and pushing away responsibilities.

Rebellious Teenagers are the black sheep of the family—love 'em or hate 'em, they do things their way. They will figure things out . . . when they're ready. And please don't try to tell them what to do. They won't be bossed around and won't take orders (which is why they have a hard time keeping a steady job). Rebellious Teenagers tell everyone that they are "survivors," and when you look at their pasts, you will, without exception, find trauma and tragedy that have befallen them. When grown, they are nothing more than dysfunctional, disempowered adults still acting like angry teenagers, who consistently sabotage their own happiness and success.

Rebellious Teenagers are emotionally stunted adults who revert back to their juvenile antics whenever they don't get their way. Always in some kind of trouble, the Rebellious Teenagers wish they could be calm, content, and easygoing, but they can't be. They can't even be on time for anything. Being late is expected—a blatant disregard of other people's time (it's not on purpose). They are angry! In fact, they are actually mad at you when *they* arrive late.

*"How dare you question me?! Do you know what I went through trying to get here?"*

But don't worry: Rebellious Teenagers always have a long conga line of Parent Archetypes enabling them by cleaning up their messes, covering up for them, and offering excuses for their behavior. But it's usually not until something serious—such as hitting rock bottom or getting a DUI—that Rebellious Teenagers even consider cleaning up their lives. They don't have to. Someone will always bail them out.

### The Troublemaker

Somehow, someway, the Troublemakers have this way of involving themselves in everyone's business; stirring the pot is their specialty! A little too nosy and opinionted for their own good, Troublemakers think nothing of disclosing information whenever or wherever they feel like it or carelessly disregarding other people's feelings by making hurtful and unnecessary comments.

What's worse is they don't just share information, they offer their extra two cents, sometimes even embellishing situations to be worse than they are. Presenting their opinions and unsolicited advice, while asking the most personal and inappropriate questions, Troublemakers pretend to be concerned about what's been happening in your life, but under their busybody demeanor are people who enjoy gossiping, while feeling somewhat superior to the people they judge and talk about.

The truth is, Troublemakers don't mean to be nasty or intrusive. Most often they don't even know how they always find themselves in the middle of the excitement—people just tell them things, and they are simply sharing what they've heard! They prefer to call themselves "networkers"—someone who knows everyone and so, of course, also seems to know the "latest news"! It's not their fault! *Besides, if you didn't want it repeated, you shouldn't have told them!*

If these individuals could expand their Emotional Edge just a little more, they would see that the same effort it takes to share negativity could be used for sharing positive things, events, and trends. These people could actually be "movers and shakers" in this world—Light Connectors! (You'll read more about this "career strategy" in Chapter Eight.)

Instead, Troublemakers—specializing in sugarcoated hostility—are well-camouflaged ringleaders who sabotage others without the gull to be direct. This would be the archetype that stoops so low as to play people (family members or friends) against one another in order to cover their own behinds. They tamper with relationships and somehow successfully make others out to be the bad guys. *Oh, it's all in fun*, they'll insist. *You're being too sensitive! They mean no harm!*

And they probably don't mean any harm . . . but they do harm. A lot.

Let's be honest, life can be difficult enough on its own; no one needs meddlesome people provoking us. We would rather avoid unnecessary trouble, and the easiest way to do that often comes down to avoiding the ones causing the trouble. Unless Troublemakers wise up, they're always going to be creating chaos in some way, shape, or form—just for the fun of it. Once you've seen Troublemakers' true colors, believe it!

### The Drama Queen

Drama, drama, and more drama! The Drama Queens desperately want attention but depend upon chaos and dysfunction because they don't know how to receive attention in a healthy way. Drama Queens are quite different from Scared Children, who are always fearful, confused, and helpless; Drama Queens can be fabulous—funny, sweet, kind, and extremely entertaining!—but they can also be full-blown divas at times!

Their Academy Award–winning performances border on super-cute, super-demanding, super-difficult, or super-spoiled! When things don't go their way, Drama Queens feel sorry for themselves, moping around the house, crying in bed, complaining about their injustices, or kicking up a temper tantrum; they want what they want, when they want it. Period. They want to create and sustain success in their lives—relationships, friendships, career, and family—but someone always ends up doing something to them. It's rarely their fault. They swear they hate drama! It just somehow follows them around.

It's just that they are the eternal actors who want nothing more than to be loved and approved of. But in the end, their complicated personalities push everyone away. You just can't please them! Nothing is ever good enough. The highs and lows are too much to take!

Super-sensitive to their own needs, Drama Queens can be insensitive to others—unaware of how difficult or demanding they can be, every conversation somehow finds a way back to them. Saying and doing inappropriate things and accepting inappropriate behavior, they've learned that if they yell loud enough or whine long enough, they'll get their way. Crying. Texting. Calling. Over and over and over and over. Then, as quickly as "the crazy" comes on, it turns off. They're back to their cute, adorable selves. Asking for forgiveness, they tilt their heads down and look up at you through those puppy-dog eyes while waiting for the storm to pass. They've gotten their dose of drama—their "fix"—so they settle down for a while.

As much as the Drama Queens are smart, witty, and sometimes incredibly fun, this archetype is ultimately disempowered. Perhaps drama initially allows them to manipulate relationships and to get the attention they need, but Drama Queens often destroy the very things they want most: love, commitment, and devotion.

### The Charmer

Charismatic, fun, sexy, and lighthearted, the Charmers have mastered the art of manipulation! Whether it's receiving gifts, jobs, opportunities, or adventures, Charmers have this amazing way of getting their needs met without having to put in the work, time, finances, or effort that others do. It's not that they don't have the talent to maintain their opportunities, they somehow can charm just about anyone into giving them what they want. They even know how to get away with breaking the rules, while giggling or winking afterward. *No harm intended!*

Man or woman, what is this power they possess?

Using body language, facial expressiveness, lighthearted vocabulary, and even sexual prowess to emphasize just how enthralled they are with you, Charmers are skilled at making you feel so important that, before you know it, you've fallen into their magical web of seduction.

Charmers have learned how to show an *exaggerated* interest in you in order to get their needs met! Skilled in verbal and nonverbal communication, never breaking eye contact, Charmers will bat their eyelashes, laugh at all your jokes, and make you feel like the most important person in the room. Charmers are great at reading people and can quickly figure out a way to get close with the person in charge, whether it's through overt flattery, subtle compliments, affirmation, or some other technique—even sex, if need be.

Fluent in the power of persuasion, they communicate their charm in the way they dress, talk, walk, dance, and move. From a sexy glance to a cute smile, Charmers exude sex appeal in all that they do and will use it, if necessary.

The downfall is that the Charmers have a hidden agenda: they are using you. The interest and attention are fake and false. The relationship will never go anywhere unless you keep giving, doing, spending, and helping them. The minute you need something in return, you'll realize Charmers aren't really that interested in you at all. They're simply interested in what you can do for them.

Eventually, after the Charmer in your life has soaked up all your energy and possibly your resources, too—taken over your client list, schmoozed with all your friends, and worked their way past your social status, only to forget you existed—it becomes much easier to see what's really going on; sadly, we often feel angry with ourselves once they skip town! (And they will move on!) Feeling used and abused, we ask ourselves, "Why did I allow myself to get sucked into this manipulation?"

Don't take it personally, Charmers never meant to hurt you. This is simply the way they've learned to get by in life. They aren't bad people; they're just beguiling!

If only these Casanovas could expand their Emotional Edge and focus on giving, caring, and enriching the lives of others rather than just mooching from and sponging off them, Charmers could be amazing Light Workers (again, we'll talk more about this "career strategy" in Chapter Eight).

### The Joker

*"Keep the good times rolling!"* Jokers are the class clowns—the comedians who try hard to keep everyone in good spirits. They are the hit at every party! Nonstop entertainers, they are quick-witted and have the gift of gab. Keeping things light is their specialty, even if that means making nonstop fun of themselves.

Your time with a Joker will never run short of laughter since this archetype knows how to keep the atmosphere light and playful. Wildly loved by most because of their dynamic nature, friendships with Jokers are sincerely valued since these individuals add so much positivity to our lives. Unfortunately, having mature, loving, "grown-up" relationships with them can prove difficult—especially if you're looking for intimacy!

The challenge with Jokers is that they don't like deep or

emotionally "heavy" conversations. Not because they aren't intelligent or thoughtful enough, but because the notion of an intimate, personal discussion paralyzes them. When it's time to get serious, they just can't. They prefer to distract, change the topic, and find something else to kid about. Seeing as they haven't learned how to address touchy or emotional situations without the assistance of joking, it's challenging to expand your relationship with the Joker from "a good time to a lifetime."

Most people translate Jokers' approach as though they aren't taking them or their feelings seriously, which can provoke the very opposite emotion of joy and laughter. You may end up feeling hurt or angry! (There isn't much else that can stir up anger quite like someone treating your vulnerable emotions as comical.)

If only Jokers could grow up just a little, they could embody the Adult Archetype so effortlessly; these people could be major Light Workers in the world because, at their core, they really are so "light and lively."

### The Warrior

Strong, fearless, and determined, the Warriors are able to convince almost everyone they are truly empowered. But don't let that tough and impenetrable exterior fool you! This archetype has its own Achilles' heel: If you dare try to cross them, warriors will blaze through relationships, even opportunities, before they ever have a chance to blossom. Aggressiveness is their "go-to" defense mechanism.

Although Warriors never look for trouble, when cornered they become the fiercest of all the archetypes. They will never start a fight, but they *will* finish one . . . right to the death of the relationship!

This archetype goes through life wearing a suit of armor

that few can pierce; they assume they must fight, claw, and force their way to the top. Nothing comes easily, but that won't stop them. They're prepared for battle at all times. The Warriors assume life is hard. They assume there is *not* enough to go around, and therefore they must compete and even annihilate their rival in order to get their needs met. It's not that Warriors aren't sweet or fun or spiritual, but when a battle approaches, they go into warrior mode. Worrying is *not* part of their behavioral repertoire! Annihilating the worry is their primary concern. You will not hurt them! Don't bother trying.

When a confrontation is on the horizon, think twice before you decide to attack! The Warriors will not hesitate to slice your esteem with little effort or empathy. They maintain an extensive knowledge of your wounds, so if you threaten them, it will become a battle you can't win. They will go in for the kill.

Equipped with an ability to slice through almost anyone with a stern glare and, if needed, a sword of words— "word*swords*words"—Warriors can take you down with a verbal assault that penetrates straight into your heart!

These driven individuals, who want better and who believe they deserve better, are often strong, motivated, focused, and loyal beyond measure to those on their team. They know that with hard work and determination they can achieve their goals. And as long as they are winning, they feel amazing about themselves and about life.

The trouble erupts into anger when they find themselves losing—which happens from time to time. When winning is what matters most, losing becomes a heavy burden for Warriors to carry.

*What happens when someone younger, faster, stronger, or better steps onto the court? What happens when Warriors can no longer compete?*

It is here, in these fearful moments, when Warriors' virility is called into question that aggression flies into action. Forgetting that all relationships have to be a "win–win" negotiation, Warriors become singularly focused on one objective: winning. Emotionally, they've been known to hurt the people they love the most. Their words are hard to forget. Not to mention, Warriors will fight until the end!

### The Narcissist

The Narcissists are people who genuinely believe that what is best for them is what's best for everyone around them, and they are incapable of confronting the discrepancies between their internal world and reality. Naturally, they assume that everyone is as interested in them as they are! *Why wouldn't you want to hear about their lives, their ideas, their dreams, their successes, etc.?* It is so much more interesting than your own!

Sadly, Narcissists don't realize that others are not simply an extension of them; they truly believe the rest of us exist to meet their needs. They may initially make us believe that they care about us, but in truth, it's quite the contrary: they care only about themselves and how we can adore and serve them. The worst part is they don't see how self-absorbed they are.

Promises, plans, and great ideas are all part of their most honest intentions, but if you're constantly feeling like you're waiting around for a friend or family member to get back to you, you're probably dealing with a Narcissist.

Sure—they don't hesitate to promise the world to you, they just rarely deliver. Half the time, they've forgotten about you entirely. The really frustrating part is that these people don't understand how their careless and reckless disregard of you is an overt form of aggression. It's hurtful!

When they aren't overlooking plans they've made with you,

they're canceling. And if they haven't canceled, they're waltz-ing in late with some fantastical reason (and don't take it per-sonally when they must leave early, as well); Narcissists always have something or somewhere else they must get to! They'd love you to believe that they are such a VIP. *"Balancing all that they have to do is just so overwhelming, even for the most organized!"*

Truth be told, they're not all that forgetful, absentminded, or overbooked (although that's what they'd hope you'd be-lieve). Narcissists can't be bothered sticking to their com-mitments, but they would never admit to that, so they play a carefree, roll-with-the-punches, super-successful, kind of act.

Don't be too hard on yourself: Narcissists are brilliant at making everything about them, insisting that you are just way too needy!

As a friend of mine once said to describe the Narcissist in her life, "They swallow up all the air in the room. You feel like you disappear when they're around." Try not to take it personally; it isn't about you. Narcissists have unreasonable ex-pectations and porous boundaries, which manifest as a sense of entitlement and even the tendency to exploit.

The frustrating part for those who love or care about Narcissists is how easily they find unsuspecting victims who willingly stroke their wounded egos, tend to their needs, and supply them with nonstop attention, which makes self-awareness and self-healing impossible. Just think of most ce-lebrities who don't have to change, improve, or evolve because they have a posse of people who cater to their self-absorbed needs and delusions.

Like all the Emotional Sub-Archetypes, if only Narcissists could expand their Emotional Edge and rise above the lower levels of communication, this archetype could be a powerful influencer in the world!

■

Those who embody the Child Archetype are overwhelmed with their emotions; some call these individuals selfish, but they really don't mean to be. If only they could manage their fear of never knowing if their future is safe, they would feel far less frenetic and overwhelmed. By learning how to set healthy boundaries and how to stop creating drama, the Child Archetype could easily ascend into the Adult and stand calmly, gently, and fully empowered in the face of the storm. In fact, if they could embody a little more of what the Parent Archetype is here to teach us about selflessness, compassion, patience, giving, caring, nurturing, and ultimately about sacrifice, the Child could expand his or her Emotional Edge and live with more faith, forethought, and freedom.

In the meantime, the Child can't help it. Something has happened to stunt them emotionally. They don't want to grow up. Maybe becoming the Adult scares them?

## THE ADULT ARCHETYPE

The highest or greatest expression of who we are (and the ideal place to be on the Empowerment Spectrum), the Adult Archetype can give and receive love equally, care for and be cared for, and give and take in all the right amounts. They are empowered, confident, kind, self-assured, and wise! The Adult Archetype has taken the journey, walked the path, done the work, healed the wounds, and they're on the road to peace. Their life is reflecting this inner peace and joy. They are in the flow! They're on the Emotional Edge: The perfect balance of following and honoring their own path, while maintaining the commitments they've made to others.

With a full ascendance of the Parent Archetype and the

Child Archetype, the Adult Archetype embodies the noblest aspects of our selfishness and selflessness, aka the Self. It is a balancing act, but the Adult innately knows how to maintain it.

Of all the books I've ever read on the concept of Self, I was most moved by Michael A. Singer's *The Untethered Soul*: "There is nothing more important to true growth than realizing you are not the voice of the mind—you are the one who hears it."

He goes on to say:

> True personal growth is about transcending the part of you that is not okay and needs protection. This is done by constantly remembering that you are the one inside that notices the voice talking. That is the way out. The one inside who is aware that you are always talking to yourself about yourself is always silent. It is a doorway to the depths of your being.

This silent witness is what I think of as the Self or the Real Me—the fully embodied, transcended, empowered Adult Archetype. For me, this is where my Woman Energy resides.

When you embody the Adult Archetype, you have fully integrated your child and parent characteristics and transcended to a new, more empowered point. You communicate with energy, enthusiasm, and joy, while maintaining composure, reason, and interdependence. You are accepting, open-minded, and willing to share yourself completely and wisely. You are autonomous and at ease in a committed relationship because you have confidence in yourself!

The Adult Archetype savors the playful, lighthearted passion love brings to one's life. They want their partners to be their "own person," with their own ideas, dreams, and hobbies:

two healthy people coming together in the spirit of harmony, unity, love, pleasure, and happiness.

The Adult Archetype is able to give and receive abundance, support, encouragement, pleasure, joy, peace, and acceptance without guilt, fear, shame, or manipulation. They are able to set and maintain healthy boundaries. They are not about perfection or achievement, but rather self-actualization, including the betterment of all. The Adult Archetype embodies the expression "Live and let live!" Although they aren't afraid to get involved when the situation calls for it, they are comfortable letting other people do things their own way.

The Adult Archetype honors the Self in body, mind, and spirit by staying connected, aware, clear, and conscious of their feelings and emotions. Their body is their messenger—their vehicle for *being*—for living, loving, moving, giving, and receiving. It is their temple. They take good care of themselves by eating nutritiously, exercising, drinking high-quality water, and getting high-quality fresh air. They know that play and laughter are essential to their lives, and they are mindful to fit in relaxation, rejuvenation, and fun!

Sexually, the Adult Archetype is aware of maintaining the balance between "you" and "me." In other words, pleasure is the modus operandi. Free of shame, guilt, fear or judgment, the Adult Archetype engages in mutually beneficial and personally enjoyable, consenting sex. They feel free and yet safe.

Mentally, the Adult Archetype knows that what they think about, they can bring about. They are confident in their abilities to devise a goal and execute it well. They understand the power of their thoughts, beliefs, and, ultimately, their emotions.

The Adult Archetype is comfortable within the world.

They see the bigger picture and are aware of global struggles, concerns, and challenges. They feel as though they are following their purpose and passion, contributing to the collective consciousness in a powerful way.

The Adult Archetype is within all of us; now we just have to bring it forth.

■

In the next few chapters, you will learn how to expand from the Parent or the Child Sub-Archetypes into the Adult Archetype by raising your level of consciousness and improving your communication skills.

A huge part of sustaining your empowerment is recognizing when you feel yourself contracting into the smallness of any of the Emotional Sub-Archetypes. Remember, whether it's The Addict (as an example), who pours another drink even though alcohol is destroying her relationships or The Micromanager who sweats the small stuff and drives everyone around him crazy with his continual "looking over your shoulder," you formed your Emotional Sub-Archetype to protect you until you felt safe enough to be your Self.

Unfortunately, over time these archetypes begin to hold us captive "in our clay," so to speak. They become the "devil on our back." The most frustrating part is that the angrier we get at them for destroying certain aspects of our life, the more disempowered we become; misdirected fear and anger annihilate us.

In Chapter Five, we will finalize the healing process by integrating your Emotional Sub-Archetypes. Integration will allow you to reach a level of self-love you've perhaps never experienced before.

As the beloved Maya Angelou, one of the most empowered

women the world has ever known, wrote "When you know better, you do better." You'll soon know better. It's then *up to you* to do better. Once you know, you know. What matters now is that you embrace the idea that *you can choose* who you want to be. You have the strength to climb the Empowerment Spectrum.

> This is crucial information:
> You have the power to decide who you will be.
> You have the power to think for yourself!

# CHAPTER THREE

# The Communication Scale

"THINK"

> Let's not forget that the little emotions are the
> great captains of our lives
> and we obey them without realizing it.
>
> VINCENT VAN GOGH

In this chapter we're focusing on the second aspect of the Empowerment Spectrum: the Communication Scale.

Our ability to communicate is the easiest indicator of our Emotional Age. But communicating our true needs can be incredibly difficult, and many of us fall into unhealthy and self-limiting patterns and behaviors. Some people are afraid to ask directly for what they need, and they adopt passive-aggressive methods rather than being honest. Other people demand what they want so aggressively that they lose the ability to connect and inevitably, they rob themselves of their own needs and desires.

Tons of books have been written on the importance of good communication, on the language of love, on how to be a good parent, and on smart ways to negotiate in business. These are all shades of what I call Empowered Communication. Based on speaking and listening in a "win-win" way, this method of communicating is crucial for your happiness and success.

The trouble is, few of us witnessed Empowered Communication while growing up—where the goal is a comfortable exchange between people who are able to express themselves freely and to find a place where both their needs are met.

Empowered Communication is the most important aspect of all relationships—including the one we have with ourselves. But it can't occur unless we are emotionally empowered—feeling good from within, that is, having peace of mind.

The truth is, if we have emotional baggage dragging us down, preventing us from stepping into our power, we can't possibly sustain a happy, empowered life; the effort of carrying around all that unfinished business and tending those old wounds is too exhausting.

Unhealed experiences keep triggering us into disempowered emotional places, which cause us to relive the suffering. Until we heal the old stories, we will continue to find ourselves stuck in certain aspects of our lives, navigating from a disempowered Emotional Archetype. We call this "self-sabotage" (although many people may not even realize they themselves are the cause of their suffering).

Self-sabotage is a clear sign that we have repressed anger and unfinished business—those feelings that have been tucked away and never dealt with are now imploding.

The good news: there are gifts in every story, if we can chip away the clay and uncover the gold.

Part of the healing process is being honest with yourself about how you are communicating and showing up in the world. This takes honesty, mindfulness, and personal insight. Ask yourself: What are my default methods of pursuing my needs? What script am I following without thinking about it? What is my Dominant Emotional Archetype?

It then requires that we climb the Empowerment Spectrum, one level at a time, until we finally transcend all the Parent and Child Sub-Archetypes and become the fully embodied, empowered Adult!

The important thing to note is that you are not leaving these parts of you behind, shrouded in shame, fear, or embarrassment. You are integrating them into the "wholeness" of who you are. You are learning how to find, listen to, and then transcend these wounded aspects of yourself. We will do this together in the coming chapters.

This chapter will look at the communication skills we all use—no matter our language, gender, age, or country of origin. It is important you understand that each level of communication builds in its degree of consciousness and emotional empowerment.

Our level of consciousness is a direct reflection of how we view those around us and ourselves; it shows us how effectively we communicate our needs, and how able we are to hear and respond to the needs of others. This is not about how frequently we get what we want. As we discussed in Chapter Two, there are several Emotional Sub-Archetypes that are very successful at getting what they want, but they do so in a way that disempowers themselves and/or the people around them in damaging ways (which inevitably hurts us all anyway).

The truth is, feeling and expressing our anger is where most of us struggle, which is why "how we deal with our anger" is the game-changer. When things don't go our way or when we don't feel that our needs are being met, our Emotional Age is most often revealed. It's easy to be assertive, composed, even loving, when you aren't being provoked or triggered. But how do you respond when you feel "tested"?

> **This is the proverbial fork in the road:**
> **One way will lead you to peaceful power, while the other will take you to raging force.**

Will you rise into your authentic Adult Archetype by re-routing your fear into Empowered Communication? Will you speak your truth with fairness and forethought?

Will you slide into forceful, self-righteous aggressiveness that demands that others do it your way . . . the only way . . . the right way? Will you become offensive or defensive?

Or worse, will you fall into a passive or passive-aggressive position and become the victim?

This chapter will offer you steps to help you rise up through your anger into assertive Empowered Communication. This is where all the good stuff is!

Empowered Communication is an art that anyone can learn, but it requires courage, honesty, personal insight, self-reflection, and the willingness to raise your level of consciousness; to manage your emotions; and to heal old wounds that keep triggering you to behave and react in old, unhealthy, disempowered ways.

Let's begin by looking first at the lower levels of the Communication Scale: Passive Communication . . .

# Passive Communication

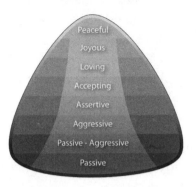

As you will learn in this section, "passive" and "peaceful" are on opposite ends of the spectrum. They represent the full range of duality or contrast within each of us. Women, in particular, need to learn this important difference.

I will admit that for most of my life, I believed my soul wanted only peace. And while this is true (our soul does want peace), what I didn't understand was the difference between Peaceful Communication and Passive Communication.

As a younger woman, when I found myself in a situation with someone I assumed was an aggressor, instead of finding my internal high road—neutral ground—I would feel my throat tightening, my chest constricting, my pulse racing, and my knees buckling. I was going into protection mode—fight or flight.

I believed that for every action there was an equal and opposite reaction, and I didn't want to fight. So without fail, something inside would whisper to me, "Take the high road, Crystal. Keep the peace. It's not worth it."

At the time, I thought "taking the high road" meant backing down or walking away, which I often did. But that was not the "high road." The path of least resistance that I trod so often was actually the "middle of the road," maybe even the "low road."

I had to learn what the "high road" actually looked like, sounded like, and felt like in my own body.

After years of "turning the other cheek" and ignoring my own needs or negating my worth, I discovered that peace isn't about everyone being the same, thinking the same, or feeling the same. It isn't even about everyone liking you or agreeing with you. Peace is honoring our differences and doing our best to find common ground. Peace is "acceptance" expanded. But you can't have peace if you're afraid to speak. You can't have peace if you're afraid to listen. Passivity, on the other hand, depends upon your fear of speaking up or disagreeing, while avoiding any kind of confrontation becomes your primary concern.

We will talk more about Peaceful Communication in the next chapter!

## THE ESSENCE OF PASSIVE COMMUNICATION

Passive Communication appears as a sense of powerlessness. We have feelings of shame, guilt, blame, hopelessness, apathy, humiliation, embarrassment, despair, inadequacy, loneliness, and sadness. We feel stuck. We are overwhelmed, unaware of how to escape the stress we're going through. Many women, in particular, have been trapped here. This is where we see archetypes such as the Wallflower, the Martyr, the Scared Child, and the Addict.

Passive Communication leaves you feeling taken advantage

of, misunderstood, exhausted, helpless, controlled, even bullied. You'll often hear passive people say things such as "I just feel bad" . . . "If only I had done something differently" . . . or "I have no choice. There's nothing I can do." Their internal dialogue is self-defeating. They believe they have no option but to wait for someone to notice and help them. But what most people don't realize is that Passive Communication is *learned*. We weren't born this way. It is not our nature to be passive.

The two men who first revealed "learned helplessness" were Martin Seligman and Steve Maier; their experiments unfortunately involved animals and were rather disturbing:

Two dogs were put into one cage that was divided into two closed sections—one dog on each side. The dogs could see each other but couldn't get to each other.

At certain intervals, both dogs would simultaneously be given electric shocks. The only difference between the dogs was that *only one* could end the shocks for both of them by pressing a lever in his side of the cage. The other dog had no way of ending the suffering. All it could do was wait for the first dog to press the lever.

So imagine, both of these dogs would receive an equal amount of electricity surging through their bodies; however, from the perspective of the second dog, there was no way to stop the pain. Both dogs were then placed together in another cage that was divided into two sections by a short partition the dogs could easily jump over. In other words, escaping the shocks would be easy for both of them.

Here's where the research was startling: the dog that had previously learned to stop the shock by pressing the lever had no problem jumping over the wall when the shocks began. The other dog, however, did not even try to escape. It did not follow its companion to physical freedom. Instead, it lay there—whining and moaning and enduring the electricity—while the other dog waited safely on the other side. Relief was one jump away, and yet the second dog suffered no matter how many times the first dog would jump to freedom.

The experiment was done over and over with different dogs. The results were the same. What is even more interesting is that the dogs that learned to be helpless responded to the same antidepressant medications that depressed people do. Once they were being treated, the medicated animals soon started to behave much like the healthy, nonmedicated dogs.

These poor animals had somehow convinced themselves that being helpless *once* means being helpless *always*—no matter what the situation. This is how quickly learned helplessness occurs. This is the reason animal trainers in the circus can chain a ten-thousand-pound elephant to a tiny rope and feel confident the animal will never try to get away. It was taught when young that escape is impossible and that to try would be futile. The elephant has formed a belief.

## TRANSCENDING THE PASSIVE

Psychologists believe this pattern of learned helplessness is similar to depression in humans. Passive people believe that they are powerless because they have been so in the past; just like the dogs in the learned-helplessness experiments, some people were taught that there is no point in trying to change their circumstances and have long since stopped trying. They feel defeated. Stuck. "Just give up. Escape is impossible. You have no choice."

But here is the exciting news: *You do not have to remain passive—feeling unimportant, unprotected, or uncertain!*

It is completely possible to take back control in your life, to feel as though you and your needs matter (because they do)!

As it turns out, the difference between people who feel permanently helpless after a bad event and those who don't rests in how they *think* about the event and whether they make the event mean something bad about them or not.

Asking questions such as "Did I cause this? Is it my fault? Does what I want even matter? Is this one event going to affect every area of my life? Am I ever going to find peace of mind?" can leave you feeling helpless long term.

The secret is to learn how to ask yourself more empowered questions that encourage you to rise above the situation and to see it through more neutral, impartial, and reasonable lenses. In order to do that, you need to look at each situation in your life as a separate incident, and not as part of a longer chain of inevitable disappointments, injuries, failures, or injustices. You also must stop seeing yourself as an extension of anyone else, whether it's with your parents, partner, children, coworkers, pets, etc. You are your own person with your own needs, dreams, and desires. You, alone, matter.

One of the most important questions I will ask myself is this: "If I weren't afraid, what would I do?"

This question allows your own inner desires and wisdom to guide you toward a more empowered future, rather than staying stuck in the past, believing what was.

The truth is, once you know, you know! Once you know what you would do if you weren't afraid, you instantly shift into a more emboldened emotional place called desire. Denying your desire will keep you stuck in passivity—learned helplessness.

Your passion must be fulfilled in order for you to be empowered, and to resonate as the Adult. But you can't find peace of mind if you aren't following your own inner light! Besides, the only way to lift the planet to its highest good is for each of us to lift ourselves to our highest good. Our happiness empowers happiness in others. We are connected to each other!

The trouble is, when we've been neglected, abused, ignored, and so on, we struggle on the deepest level with knowing our own worth and accepting that we were born to be happy. Perhaps we believe what they've said about us and now we negate ourselves, too. We feel ashamed of who we are. Our energy goes into trying to convince the world (and maybe even ourselves) that we are good enough. Eventually, we run out of energy with all this performing and proving. It's inauthentic and exhausting. Passivity sets in. Despair. Depression.

In the international bestselling book *Think and Grow Rich*, Napoleon Hill insisted that a burning desire is the root of all achievement.

By focusing on your desires rather than on past letdowns, you redirect your thoughts toward possibilities rather than problems. Besides, if you don't achieve your desires, frustration will then set in! And that's okay! It's natural! Normal! Even necessary!

Anger and frustration are more empowered than apathy and hopelessness, which is why anger is a necessary emotion on the way to empowerment! Anger is simply a "stepping stone"!

The secret is to give your anger a *healthy* voice—a safe place for its expression, recognition, and ascension. Anger is occurring because something doesn't feel tolerable and you are being asked to deal with it. It is showing up because there is limiting belief *in you* that must be acknowledged, accepted, and recontextualized in a way that will allow for you to get your needs met. Denying your anger will keep you stuck in Passive-Aggressive Communication.

## Passive-Aggressive Communication

As we shift up out of Passive Communication, we move into emotions of fear, desire, and frustration, which are the driving forces behind Passive-Aggressive Communication. Many of the Child and the Parent Sub-Archetypes fall into this style of interacting, negotiating, and trying unsuccessfully to compromise. Rarely is long-term success seen in this level of consciousness because there is still too much struggle, shame, and blame, that is, repressed anger!

The real problem for both the Passive-Aggressive Communicators and those who are trying to interact with them is that you can never have a truly honest and open relationship with these folks. They simply don't (or can't) say what they *really* mean and they don't mean what they say.

Truth be told, they don't always realize how indirect and roundabout their communication style is. Passive-Aggressive Communicators may not even realize how little self-advocacy they are doing. They've spent a lifetime being let down, abused, or ignored. They swing between trying to be what you want them to be and wanting you to try to figure out who they really are. There is a lot of fear in this communication zone!

Ever heard the saying, "What you fear, you draw near"? These folks are so afraid of not being accepted, loved, or not having their needs met that instead of sharing their feelings in a fair, solution-oriented, "win-win" way they find subtler ways to let you know they aren't happy—making sarcastic jokes and little digs, uttering antagonistic comments, asking inappropriate questions, whining, complaining, blaming, gossiping, making snippy remarks, pretending to be less capable than they are (that is, playing dumb), procrastinating, or deliberately or repeatedly failing to complete requested tasks for which they're responsible; even stubbornness, bitterness, and sullenness can be seen as passive-aggressive.

*Maybe this has been you?*

Have you reverted to pouting, slamming doors, mumbling under your breath, or throwing snarky remarks in the direction of someone you're frustrated with?

*Of course you have! We all have!*

Most of us have little idea of what to do with our fear, anger, and frustration—especially women. We were taught to bury our unhappiness. Women should never demand what they want and should certainly not express displeasure if they don't get it. Unhappy women are unlikable. Shameful.

Culturally, men can have "an edge," and it's considered manly, even sexy. But being an edgy woman is unacceptable, inappropriate, and improper; even the Bible says so: "It is better to live in a desert land than with a contentious and vexing woman" (Proverbs 21:19). And so we try to hide our anger. Cover it. Nullify the fact that under the surface there are a lot of injustices. In my family, children were to be seen and not heard. We were not allowed to express any emotions other than happiness, gratitude, and niceties.

We kids were taught that what goes on in our house, stays in our house; that no matter what your parents do, you are not to talk back, be disobedient, or *tell a soul.* Not to mention, speaking to a therapist, psychologist, or pastor was for losers. The weak needed therapy. The weak needed God. Religion was a crutch, my father told us.

In fact, I distinctly remember being about seventeen, homeless, and taking the city bus alone to the hospital for treatment on my cervix. Afterward, I went to visit my maternal grandmother. She asked me questions about my mom, as she hadn't heard from her daughter in a while, either. I was minimalizing the situation; sharing as much as I felt was appropriate because I knew secrets are secrets. That's when I told Grandma that I could forget but I couldn't forgive my mother for abandoning, betraying, and neglecting my siblings and me. She told me that I had to forgive my mom—the Ten Commandments said so. She opened the Bible and read it to me. I felt incredibly confused. Part of me knew this commandment was true and right and yet, it didn't align with my personal sensibilities. I was angry, hurt, and sad. I had no idea how to forgive my mother, especially when I was still enduring her abuse. I couldn't figure out why no one in my family would get involved. Everyone was afraid. For goodness sake, my little sister was only ten years old and needed someone other than just me to be her advocate. Nevertheless, I did everything in my power to be a good daughter, a good sister, and eventually, a good wife. Shut up and put up! I'd basically been told. Clearly, the legacy ran deep.

Perhaps, you, too, struggle with being honest about your true feelings. I understand if it's difficult for you to acknowledge your needs, especially if you've spent a lifetime suppressing them or being told they don't matter. Maybe, it's even more difficult for you to express your needs, so I know that it can be tempting to fall into pouting or other passive-aggressive behaviors to let other people know that you're not happy. But you have to start somewhere; you have to force yourself out of your comfort zone to start communicating in a healthier way.

Having the Emotional Edge is an ownership of desires, entitlement of expression, and permission to advocate for one's self, even in the face of conflict.

Truth be told, it is not until you finally desire empowerment enough that empowerment can occur, which means it's
okay to have an edge!

> It's the edge that gives us the contrast to decide that we
> are ready to soar in our lives! It's the same edge of the
> ever-expanding universe—the horizon line of possibility—
> that will be expanding forever for the empowered, enabled
> person!

If you've been in a passive position, rising up into Passive-
Aggressive Communication is natural and normal. You're getting closer to the edge. It's not okay, however, for you to stay
stuck on the edge! It reminds me of the beautiful poem written
by Christopher Logue:

> *Come to the edge.*
> *We might fall.*
> *Come to the edge.*
> *It's too high!*
> *COME TO THE EDGE!*
> *And they came,*
> *and he pushed,*
> *and they flew.*

When you feel as though you are soaring in your life, you
know you have expanded your Emotional Edges!

## THE ESSENCE OF PASSIVE-AGGRESSIVE COMMUNICATION

The trouble is that most passive-aggressive people have a
deep fear of facing themselves, and this means they will have

a challenging time looking for solutions from within! They come just to the edge, complain a lot, backtrack, and repeat the pattern over and over again.

If this is you, I understand that navigating your life from this place is a protection mechanism to prevent you from being hurt. You're afraid! Sharing your needs and feelings hasn't proven to be a positive experience for you. Operating from one of the Emotional Sub-Archetypes feels safer than stepping *fully* into your power!

Perhaps, you're hoping someone or something will help heal you. Maybe, you want others to know you well enough to be able to read your mind and anticipate your needs. The trouble is that you are also afraid of opening yourself up completely, and so you have rarely felt entirely connected to anyone. You give just enough to have a relationship but then pull away or start testing other people before you have the chance to develop a strong bond. You sabotage things. *The worst part is that you know you're sabotaging but you don't know how to do it differently.*

We've all heard the definition of insanity: Doing the same thing over and over and expecting different results. And yet, you keep playing the same "theme song" over and over in your life, expecting a different ending!

Until you get healthy, your relationships won't be healthy.

The reason most of us find ourselves stuck is because we're holding out for things to get better, and yet at the same time we're afraid that they never will. We're afraid of change. We're afraid to let go. We're afraid of the unknown. We're in pain, suffering in denial. We're lost. We desperately cling on, trying to control the outcome, manipulating things as we're navigating in the dark.

The real problem is that we resist "the dark"—the unhappy, scary, or negative feelings we've buried deep—because we think we can't deal with it, without becoming disempowered. So afraid of what might surface if we allow feelings such as shame, guilt, apathy, sadness, fear, or anger to come up, most of us will do almost anything not to let them out. We find ways to grab, hold, and contain them—excessive eating, drinking, smoking, shopping, working, gambling, exercising, rescuing, arguing, complaining, saving, volunteering, even troublemaking.

It's as though we build a dam around our heart and do our best to hold everything in. But passive aggressiveness begins when those "bad" feelings have been bottled up for so long that our wall begins to crack. All those pent-up emotions start squirting out in places where we didn't intend to manifest them, or in little ways that leave everyone feeling unsettled.

In order to transcend Passive-Aggressive Communication, we must tear down the wall, piece by piece, and allow *all* our emotions to exist. And here's a secret: when we aren't working so hard to bottle the bad ones up, our emotions are not really that overwhelming! Rather than the tidal wave that we're afraid of, emotions can be simple ripples on the water that we acknowledge but are not overwhelmed by.

## Transcending Passive-Aggressive Communication

The Passive-Aggressive Communicator needs to establish trust that their ideas are valid and will be heard. In other words, trust that you *deserve* to be listened to, protected, and respected. If you're in an environment where this is not the case—where you do not feel safe—it is not your fault, whether or not you allowed it! Self-shaming and living with guilt will not empower you to make the changes you need to make. Instead, you need to find a safe place to learn how to begin expressing yourself, your feelings, and your needs. But it all begins with you. *You have to give yourself permission to matter!* Believe it or not, the most dynamic, successful, happy people have mastered self-advocacy with generosity!

One of the primary differences between the lower communication levels and the higher communication levels is the way that we deal with feelings of shame, guilt, apathy, sorrow, fear, desire, and anger.

Shame says, "Who I am is no good."

Guilt says, "What I did is no good."

Apathy says, "I feel stuck. Nothing ever changes or gets better."

Sorrow says, "This is *not* how it is supposed to be."

Fear says, "I'm afraid to go back to what was and even more afraid of the unknown."

Desire says, "I know there's something better out there . . ."

Anger says, "This is no longer acceptable!"

For many of us, the rumbling anxiety of fear is too much to bear, so instead of rising up through it—facing it and finding the gold in it—we find a way to stuff all our unhappy thoughts and misdirected worries back down. Paralysis analysis. We numb out. Mindless.

Here is what you must know: nothing good is going to come from suppressing, contracting, or negating your feelings—especially the "bad" ones. All that will do is impress upon you to worry more, do more, think more, stress more, and try harder. Gripping. Grasping. Clenching. Forcing. Controlling. It's like trying to submerge a huge beach ball under the surface of the water. It takes a lot of work! Eventually, you're exhausted. Helpless. Disempowered.

When you make choices and communicate from this passive-aggressive place, you can guarantee a negative outcome.

And if you think shaming, guilting, or scaring people will empower them to make better choices, you are sadly mistaken.

One simple yet profound exercise you can do for yourself is learn to "feel." *For me, learning to feel has been the single most important aspect to my empowerment.*

All your feelings reside in your body. Your body is your messenger, speaking to you 24/7. Your body tells you everything you need to know: what lights you up, what drains your life force, which foods work with your system, which emotions you're suppressing, who is good for you, and so on. Every ache, every pain, every joy, and every pleasure—whether comfortable, uncomfortable, exhausting, or energizing—your body is the outward expression of to what degree you are in alignment with your Self.

Resistance in your body is showing you that something is out of alignment; it must be healed in order for you to feel physically and emotionally empowered.

Instead of struggling with your body or numbing the pain, you need to see it as a gift, offering you an opportunity to uncover the unhealthiest or most wounded aspects of yourself that fears, judges, condemns, blames, and worries. Pain offers you a chance to transcend your suffering and step into your power!

*Why not take a moment and ask your body what it is trying to tell you?*

A great way to do this is to travel into your body, find the areas where your pain resides, and learn to dialogue with it. If you'll listen, you will never again need to diet, fear illness, or struggle with a lack of energy.

## "HEALING THE FEELING"—GUIDED MEDITATION

Let's get started:

Begin by sitting in a comfortable chair.

Back upright. Breathing deeply, right down to your belly button.

Close your eyes and give yourself a few moments to become mindful and relaxed.

Let your mind unwind. Let your shoulders drop down from your ears. Let your breathing deepen and expand.

Wonderful.

I want you to picture in your mind a "mini you" standing on a platform, similar to an elevator. When you feel ready, I want you to see yourself lowering down out of your brain and into your breath.

As you lower down out of your head—out of your brain and into your body—I want you to imagine you have a special X-ray machine that can laser in on every ache and pain from the top of your head to the tip of your toes.

Pay attention to how you feel: Is your body light, peaceful, calm, pain-free, and relaxed? Or do you have places that feel heavy, constricted, anxious, uncomfortable, ill, or injured?

Let's take a moment to travel over to your heart to ask it how open and vulnerable it feels? Take a few deep breaths and let's see what comes up for you.

Does your heart feel like a huge, happy ball of love and trust—open and expansive? Or do you feel like it is closed off, behind a wooden cabinet with a big padlock? Safe and sound. Alone. Protected.

Continue to breathe deeply and gently. Let whatever needs to come up to speak to you. Don't deny it. Nothing is off-limits. You are allowed to tell the truth—especially to yourself! You are allowed to feel.

If your heart seems closed down for business, it's okay. I understand why. You've been hurt. You're afraid. But for the next few minutes, let's try to allow your heart to expand.

Next, I want you to ask yourself how willing you are to find the key that will unlock your heart?

If you are ready, in your mind's eye, find the key in your pocket and unlock the cabinet. Remove it and put it on the table beside you.

Wonderful!

How does that feel?

Take a deep expansive breath. Inhale. Exhale.

Feel your heart and lungs opening, expanding, and receiving.

And then, let it go. Relaxing, trusting, allowing.

Take another deep breath.

Comforting, safe, free. In and out.

Allow your Self to soak and simmer in this relief . . . this safe place.

Security.

Protection.

Freedom.

How does it feel to relax? To not have to do, be, become, fix, save, rescue anyone?

Allow yourself to steep and soak in this expansive space of safety, care, and well-being.

Now, let's get back to that special X-ray machine. I want you to laser in on the areas on your body that hurt the worst. Let's travel into your pain and suffering—into the tightest or sorest spots (such as your aching back or bloated tummy), and let's dialogue with them.

Ask your body:

> If you could give this resistant feeling or painful area an emotion, what would it be called? Anger? Sorrow? Fear?
> (Breathe into the emotion. Allow it to intensify.)

Who or what is this stored emotion connected to? (Isn't it emotionally exhausting to carry this person or pain around with you?)

How long have you been holding on to this feeling?

How is holding on to this hurting you? (Allow yourself to feel the intensity of how this buried emotion is causing you physical pain and suffering.)

If you could see this person in your mind's eye, what would you want him or her to know? (Allow yourself to say everything you've needed to say. Give yourself full permission to speak your truth. Nothing is off-limits.)

Once you have said everything you need to say, I want you to imagine you have a special pair of scissors. See yourself cutting the cord between you and him or her. Watch this person or the pain he or she caused float away to Heaven/ God/the Universe/the Light/Source Energy (whatever word feels appropriate to you). This great omnipotent Presence will transmute the pain and suffering back into love and life.

I want you to allow yourself to travel back into this painful area and then, using your breath, begin to visualize yourself breathing "love and light" directly into the pain. On your exhale, allow yourself to draw the pain up and out of your body then blow it away. Visualize yourself letting go of the heartache this person brought to you. Allow the light to spread throughout your entire body until you feel more at ease.

**I breathe in love and light. I exhale pain and suffering.**

Continue to breathe deeply and expansively. (Conscious breathing is one of the very best ways to release fear and expand consciousness.)

Once you feel ready, bring yourself back to the room.

Your next step is to write this person a letter. This should not be a carefully worded, friendly letter that contains nothing that will offend. You're not actually going to mail it, so don't worry about spelling, grammar, or punctuation. Just write from your deepest wounds. Allow yourself to be honest with yourself about all the "should've beens," "could've beens," and "ought to have beens." Allow yourself to empty out all the "held on to" pain and suffering, because whatever is repressed will find a way to be expressed. This is a very powerful and important process for you to go through in order to find healing.

Remember, you are not going to send this letter. The person to whom you are writing doesn't need to read the letter for this exercise to work! But if you can, I want you to share your letter with someone you trust. It is important for you to "name it" and "claim it."

Then, once you feel ready, your final step is to burn the letter and say good-bye. This is a crucial part of this process. I call this part "grieving it" and "releasing it." You must burn your letter.

If you don't have a wood-burning stove or fireplace, take your letter outside and place it in a lasagna pan. Light your letter and watch as the words burn away, letting go of the emotional bond the past has held over you.

Now you may be thinking, "Crystal, I thought I'd dealt with this already!"

You probably have dealt with some of it, *maybe even most of it*! But healing happens in layers—just like in that well-known onion analogy. It is a process. And if you do this work, you will get there!

For those who want to avoid this process because you believe you can avoid dealing with your buried emotions or triggers, you are mistaken. You will never find peace of mind if you continue to practice avoidance.

I've had to do this letter writing process many times regarding the same person, over the course of many years. It has helped me to be mindful of my codependency—my need to please others, while negating my own feelings—particularly with my closest loved ones, i.e. *"When you are happy, I'm happy. When you are sad, I can't be happy until I make you happy, even if it means sabotaging myself."*

When I feel myself contracting—taking on the weight of the world or the suffering of a loved one—I remind myself to mentally "cut the cord" so that I can be my own sovereign woman—loving but not attached. Light. Empowered. Emotionally healthy. This is particularly important if you struggle with "people pleasing."

(Note: As you heal one area, you may notice other aches and pains surfacing. You can redo this exercise focusing on each resistant place until your body is completely at ease. Visit me at **www.TheEmotionalEdge.com** if you would like to download my guided meditation of this process called "Healing the Feeling.")

## Facing the Fear

Something I want you to know is that facing fear is a mental game. As soon as you realize that you are infinitely more powerful than your fear is, it will never again have power over you!

You see, fear never wants you to realize how small and false it truly is because its strength lies in your believing it is stronger than it is. This is how you give your power away. This is how fear wins.

I understand the idea that facing anything negative—especially the negativity within—is scary, but let me assure you: although fear is a bastard, you can rise through it and come out the other side to a more beautiful, empowered place.

**Facing our fear is the missing piece to our finding happiness!**

Most of us have a whole gamut of buried emotions that want to rise up and come out. These buried emotions need to be freed. They've been locked inside of us (and maybe even in our family's legacy) for a long time. Facing them can be very scary!

But don't worry! Your brilliant brain will allow you to process only a layer or two at a time, so as to not allow you to become too overwhelmed or excessively flooded. If unhappy emotions come up, it's okay (Although, I know how scary it can be!). Your tears are healing. Cleansing. Releasing. Expanding.

If you've never felt immobilized by fear, let me explain how restrictive, oppressive, and constrictive it can be: fear makes sane people feel out of control and, sometimes, even as if death is imminent.

Imagine believing that something outside of you has the power to hurt you, *get you*, and take from you. So we cling to what we know, afraid to venture outside the box.

As my dad used to say, "It's better to stay with the devil you know than the devil you don't."

I'm here to tell you, he was wrong.

Your fear may try to convince you to stay where you are, suggesting that if you try to make changes, an avalanche of dark feelings will be released and nothing but bad days will await you. But *that's not true.*

Here is the most important message I want you to know:

> **Only you can choose to give your power away.**
> **Nothing or no one can take your power from you. Your strength lies in your courage to tell the truth.**

If you choose to downshift from an empowered emotional place into fear, *you've* chosen to give your power away. Most often, it is an unconscious choice driven by your limiting belief that feeling your feelings and speaking your truth is unsafe, but it is still your choice.

When we operate in fear, we feel afraid to live *fully* and to show up in the world as the greatest expression of who we are.

We may be afraid of others, afraid of their jealousy (we call it the "evil eye"), or afraid of their judgment, retribution, public attacks, even of being ostracized and unwanted.

What if they hurt us because we stand out? What if people don't like us and they say bad things about us? What if we get absolutely no support or encouragement from our friends and family and we feel even worse about ourselves—even less important?

Maybe we fear failure (that would be embarrassing), even though we've all failed so many times we should be comfortable with it by now!

Or we fear we may succeed, and what if it *really* is lonely at the top? What if no one will love us because they think *we think* we're better than them now?

What if we realize in all our success and happiness that the people in our lives are actually assholes who've been so negative and unkind to us that we no longer want to hang out with them? What then? Will we have to leave them? *Then what?*

What if we become totally fit, fabulous, healthy, wealthy, successful, and happy? What if doing so makes us selfish and self-serving?

What if we can't handle ourselves . . . because we can't trust ourselves to take care of ourselves? What if we lose control?

What if we can't trust that all will work out perfectly? What if it doesn't work out perfectly? Then what?

*I explained fear this way to my kids:*

Your fear is actually similar to a tiny mouse hiding in the basement. It scurries around in the dark, making little noises. Finally, you come down the stairs with your flashlight (your internal, blaring, bright light) and shine the light around. All you see is a monstrous dark shape in the corner, when, in fact, it is only the shadow of a tiny mouse, with your light amplifying its size and appearance.

You, terrorized by the size of the shadow, scream and run in the opposite direction, back up the stairs. You lock the basement door and get more security—maybe some big scary pit bulls and weapons.

But your fear doesn't want to be alone and rejected. It is a part of you! It belongs inside of you as much as your love and happiness do!

"Why do you keep shunning me?" it wonders. "I can't hurt you! *You* are the one hurting you! I'm here for a reason. Stop running from me!"

Eventually, your fear finds a way to get your attention again, and you get pulled back into more anxious thoughts and more surging adrenaline. And the pattern repeats itself.

**Patterns are nothing more than fearful thoughts and beliefs passed down, generation to generation.**

So the next time fear taps you on the shoulder, turn and look directly at it. Stand at the edge of the shadow. Face it. See it for what it is: a tiny mouse with *your* huge powerful light magnifying it into something it's not. It's so small compared to you!

 **If you knew your Real Self, you'd be in awe of yourself.**

The important thing to know is that fear itself is *not* an empowering emotion. It's actually quite draining. Anyone who has lived in a state of fear knows how exhausting it is. We feel like we can't shake this devil off our back. No matter what we do, our submerged fear figures out a way to resurface and then, we have to push it back down. It's grueling work!

Nevertheless, fear can take on a life of its own, making it challenging for us to separate what is true from what is exaggerated and even, possibly, completely false. Our thoughts are dark and clouded when we are in fear; our choices appear to be limited and constricting because we can't see the bigger picture while we're stuck down here in this level of communication.

It's important to remind yourself that fear serves a purpose: fear is intended to be a quick, instinctive shot of adrenaline to show you where you are contracting into a belief that isn't true and to push you back up into a more empowered place—where you are negotiating, compromising, trusting, and expressing yourself at a higher, more expansive level.

Fear, when harnessed properly, helps us pay attention to when we are about to give away our power; when, if we don't grab ahold of ourselves, we may continue to sink into the depths of despair.

We are not meant to resonate down here suffering in

silence, though, and that is why so many of us get into trouble. Prolonged exposure to these emotions can literally kill us: high blood pressure, obesity, diabetes, heart disease, cancer, stroke—the whole gamut of adrenal-based illnesses.

The trouble is, most of us do everything not to think about our fears and not to give any power to them, but there is a popular saying: "What we fear, we draw near!"

Untended fear can fester if it is ignored, feeding upon secrets, shame, guilt, and anger to stay alive. It scares us into believing that if we shine light on our limiting beliefs, painful stories, or oppressive situations, individually or globally, we will be weakened and more prone to being hurt. It depends upon us to cower and run rather than stand up and believe in ourselves, others, and in humanity. It needs us to believe that the debilitating, astringent, and suffocating feelings that may rise up within us are real and that bad things are going to happen if we reveal them and rock the boat. It depends upon us to stay small, scared, and passive.

One of the secrets to living with empowerment is facing your fear by giving it attention, kindness, and even love, that is, by letting the submerged beach ball surface!

I know this may sound counter-productive and perhaps even bizarre: *How can we send "love" to our worst enemy: fear? Why would we want to give our fear attention when all we want is to avoid it! Why would we let it out?*

Well, because love has this amazing way of healing all things.

Besides, for every action, there is an equal and opposite reaction. When we fight ourselves, we can never win! If fighting worked, we should have won the wars on terrorism, cancer, and drugs by now!

The bottom line is that fear has arrived! Just because we've figured out a way to *not feel it or to fight it* doesn't mean it will go away. It won't! It will wait as long as it needs to for us to face it and find a different way of communicating with it.

> **The only way to eradicate darkness is to shine light on it.**

There is a profound statement that, for good reason, has stood the test of time: the truth will set you free!

*The question to ask yourself in the face of unbridled fear is, "What is the truth?"*

David Ropeik, the director of risk communication at the Harvard Center for Risk Analysis in Boston, Massachusetts, wrote a compelling article on why fear has reached such epidemic proportions, blaming much of it on the Internet and media. He shares:

> Humans appear to fear similar things, for similar reasons. The study of risk perception reveals that our responses to risks are not simply internal "rational" risk analyses, but also intuitive "affective" responses that apply our emotions, values and instincts as we try to judge danger. Risk perception helps to explain why our fears often do not match the facts.

It doesn't much help matters, Ropeik points out, that we live in a world where a small majority controls what the rest of us will know.

In the United States alone, twenty-two owners decide what 70 percent of the total number of newspaper readers nationwide will read; three-quarters of American television stations are owned by only 6 percent of all media corporations.

To satisfy the need to maximize profits, risks must sound as dramatic, threatening, and urgent as possible: "Whenever something is discovered that is even possibly a peril," Ropeik writes, "we learn of it, worldwide, within hours. Word of SARS spread far faster than the disease itself."

Not to mention, anyone can publish an article on the Internet, stating information as factual when, in fact, it isn't. Just Google any symptom of illness and you will find hundreds of thousands of pages of information immediately at your fingertips: "You're going to die. You aren't going to die. You need to worry. You don't need to worry." The Information Age has overloaded us. Stress is at our fingertips 24/7.

*What does this all mean in simple terms?*

Our opinions or beliefs about ourselves, the world, and our safety in it create our fear; this helps explain why our fears often do not match the facts!

Many of our fears are the result of pure speculation about things we don't have enough information on. Once that happens we tend to fill in the gaps with scenarios that are not necessarily realistic. The bottom line is that you may get a lot of relief by assessing how realistic they are and to what degree they are based on reality.

In therapy, this approach is known as *cognitive reconstructuring*—you first identify your negative, anxiety-provoking thoughts and then start to look for evidence that could challenge these fears. Once you're connected with what you're truly feeling and fearing, you want to make sure that you're not jumping to conclusions or blowing things out of proportion. You need to see to what extent your fears are real. You want to have clarity on whether your fear is based on facts or whether your fear is just a thought.

One of the ways you can do this is to pull out your journal and ask yourself questions such as:

1. Is my reaction in proportion to the actual event?
2. What evidence is there that my fear is realistic?
3. What evidence is there that my fear might not be completely realistic?
4. What meaning am I giving to this event (remember the dogs from the experiment)?
5. Is there another way of looking at this situation?
6. If I were to look at this event from a distance what would I see?

Perhaps we must accept what the Roman philosopher Epictetus said two millennia ago: "Men are disturbed not by things, but by the view which they take of them."

Does this mean you should leave your front door wide open, inviting criminals to come in and dine with you because fear isn't real? *No!*

You must always trust your instincts and move toward higher ground. This is what it means to "take the high road." Think for yourself! Listen to your body! Protect your Self!

There were few animals killed in the horrible tsunami in 2004 that killed so many people in Sri Lanka, Thailand, India, and bordering countries. Scientists believe that's because the animals instinctively knew something was wrong, and they fled to higher ground hours in advance. The only animals killed were domesticated ones like dogs and sheep.

Allowing yourself the opportunity to *feel* is mandatory if you want to be healthy, intuitive, and empowered. You'll discover that feeling your feelings may seem scary at first, while your wounds are healing, but soon there will be little left that will trigger you to return to those old, raw, vulnerable places. You will be amazed at how quickly even the deepest wounds can heal, leaving you strong, healthy, and unblemished.

Don't let false courage and pride persuade you to not dig in and do the work of facing your fears, healing yourself, and becoming empowered! Don't be terrorized by your own shadow . . . your own fear . . . your own mind.

Remind yourself that your brain doesn't work at random. One of its biggest objectives is to ensure your survival. Your brain is far more concerned with your physical or emotional survival than it is with presenting you with an objective reality.

So from the time you were a small child you began accepting beliefs about everything from God and the devil to sicknesses you can't control to gender, sexuality, cultures, countries, and religions that are out to get you! You decided if you are lovable, important, and worthy . . . or not. You learned a whole slew of beliefs to be factual truths.

The questions you must ask yourself are these: *"How is all this working for me? Are my beliefs serving me? Is suppressing my fear healthy?"*

Those of us who have faced our stories and drawn all the shame, guilt, blame, and sorrow out of them know the struggle you might be facing when it comes to empowerment work. We call these moments (or episodes) Dark Nights of the Soul.

But in truth, your soul is never dark. It may be covered with a whole lot of clay (unneeded protection), but it is never weak, scared, ashamed, or afraid. Your *soul* is who you *really* are!

Your soul knows exactly what you need. Once you chip away all the stories (that perhaps, once served as protection), you will know how unlimited, expansive, and unstoppable you really are—you will live an empowered and fulfilling life!

Please don't let the possibility of experiencing a few dark days prevent you from finding emotional freedom and personal empowerment. It's short-term pain that will give way to long-term joy! Don't fear your fear! Don't fear your past! Don't fear your emotions! Don't fear your enemies! In fact, why don't you invite your fear of the dark basement to join you upstairs and have some fun? Maybe you'll even get a little cage for it and call it a hamster. Fear loves running on those little hamster wheels!

**Fear loses its power when you see it, talk about it, and face it!**

The events of your past have all taught you so much about who you are and who you want to be. They have taught you about empathy, compassion, and love. Your past can be the jet fuel that ignites your future happiness.

Please don't be embarrassed of yourself, your needs, or your Emotional Sub-Archetype(s). Don't be afraid you'll be shunned for unfounded fear, or that you'll be trapped forever underneath it. Just remind yourself that, as real as your fear feels, it's within your power to control it. The only monstrous thing in the room is your own light, creating that huge shadow.

Granted, those feelings you feel are certainly "real"—caused by the adrenaline pumping through your body because of the thoughts you're having—but the thoughts really aren't accurate. Disempowered thoughts are never truthful or honest. They are driven by our fear of being ostracized by our family, friends, and community. Secrets keep us hovering in shame, blame, guilt, and fear. This is what causes paralysis analysis. This is why we remain afraid. We are so embarrassed to reveal our imperfections—especially those disempowered, repetitive thoughts that distract and numb us from the real stuff.

When I feel myself not wanting to feel fear, which shows up as me trying to "numb out" through a variety of coping mechanisms from excessive working, eating, drinking, rescuing, TV watching, reading, exercising, sleeping, dieting, even creating drama, I remind myself that *if I want to heal, I have to feel—the good, the bad, and the ugly.* I know "this too shall pass." I breathe deeply. I honor myself, and whatever is surfacing. I listen, learn, and then, let it go. I feel the feeling without becoming the emotion.

## Aggressive Communication

In every situation there is an authentic (appropriate) and inauthentic (inappropriate) way to express ourselves. Aggressive Communication is the inappropriate way. It manifests in fury, rage, irrational behavior, and the annihilation of relationships. People shut up and shut down because aggressive people have no boundaries; they want *what* they want, *how* they want it, and *when* they want it. You will either agree with them or be silent. And if you disagree, get ready for the wrath of the aggressor. These folks truly believe that success only comes to those who fight hard enough for it. Someone always wins and someone always loses. That's just the way it is! Suck it up, buttercup!

Aggressive Communication shows up in any number of negative behaviors, from being self-righteous and judgmental to being difficult, demanding, cruel, argumentative, condemning, indifferent, critical, unsympathetic, insensitive, cold, careless, or simply by showing reckless disregard for another person's heart or well-being.

As I tell my daughters, you have the right to question authority, to disagree, to share your opinions, to speak up, and to speak out! But you do *not* have the right to be rude, mean, disrespectful, or belligerent. You cannot scream, rage, hit, demand, accuse, bully, undermine, hurt, damage, frighten, coerce, manipulate, threaten, or intimidate in order to get your way. And if you don't feel respected or acknowledged by someone when you're sharing your truth, you do *not* have the right to snub, humiliate, or disregard that person. Shaming is as disempowered as screaming. If someone is being inappropriate, you set a healthy boundary and walk away (in other words, when you yell at me, I feel disrespected; if you can't speak to me calmly, I'm leaving) but you do *not* engage in confrontation and you do *not* stonewall. A debate is fine and sometimes necessary, but don't let it go beyond that. If you want to be an empowered woman, raise the bar for yourself.

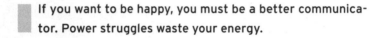

**If you want to be happy, you must be a better communicator. Power struggles waste your energy.**

Anger itself is not the problem. Truth be told, all great change has occurred because someone got angry enough to deal with an injustice. The problem comes when we are so blinded by anger that we lose sight of our ultimate goal, which is to communicate and advocate for our needs in a "win-win" way.

## THE POWER OF ANGER!

Here are the facts: You can't avoid your anger or your unhappiness. If you try to suppress it, squash it, deny it, or run from it, it will still be with you wherever you go. You'll bring your baggage into your next job, love affair, or exercise regime. It's similar to those who lose a significant amount of weight, only to gain it all back and then some. They didn't face their repetitive, fear-driven thoughts, feelings, and beliefs. They were externally focused on change rather than internally driven. Instead, they simply exchanged overeating with dieting: one oppressive condition for another.

Whatever is repressed will find a way to be expressed. Patterns continue until they're broken. You have to face yourself and your stuff. You have to dig it up and deal with it. *You have to move through it.* There is no other way. You can't go over it, under it, around it, or behind it. And you can't keep blaming all the people in your life—even if they did hurt you!

Yet, if we were to be brutally honest, anger may be the most powerful emotion many of us have ever felt. It is what spurs us on, even while it encourages our own self-importance and pride.

*This matters, dammit! You will listen to me!*

An empowered person, on the other hand, knows that anger is a natural and often legitimate emotion, but that if *held on to or misdirected*, anger destroys.

## BUT WE'RE ANGRY!

The fact is, it doesn't matter why our aggressiveness detonates; we simply can't let ourselves fly off the handle into rage or otherwise. Sometimes, aggression yields short-term results; sometimes it doesn't. But the aftershock of a blowup can have long-lasting repercussions and destroy the trust we've built with those we love. Afterward, we can't use excuses such as "I had too much to drink," "I'm PMSing," or "I'm just under too much stress! I'm sorry!"

Sorry is an important acknowledgment of wrongdoing, but only if it's accompanied by a true effort to change. Sorry doesn't cut it if you repeat the behavior over and over. And it doesn't matter if you've been wonderful for months or even years . . .

one overly aggressive attack is all it takes to end a relationship permanently or, at the very least, to damage it severely. Instead of showing respect, dignity, and healthy boundaries, we abuse our power, and our anger begins to shift into fury and, possibly, even rage. We don't acknowledge our own self-worth or that of the other person.

*This is why misdirected anger is so dangerous.*

We've all heard sayings such as this one: "You can tell the size of a man by the size of the problems that upset him."

The problem for most of us is that we are angry! But no one taught us what to do with our anger! We feel like a bottle of champagne: agitate us too much and we'll explode! Shamefully, we then jam back the cork and hope it all just simmers down on its own. But it never does. And never will. It can't without a healthy expression.

Anger, misdirected or oppressed, steals our energy, robs us of our joy, and shows the world a side of us that isn't our true Self. We'll do and say inappropriate things. We'll hurt people. We'll hurt ourselves. Most of us have no idea why we act this way or how we can channel it into something positive. We were never given the tools for doing so. For most of us, anger simply represents the "alpha," the winner, the top of the food chain.

## TRANSCENDING AGGRESSIVE COMMUNICATION

The solution is channeling our anger into Assertive Communication and, ultimately, into Peaceful Communication. This is where the Adult Archetype begins to show up.

Assertive Communication is the appropriate or authentic way to express our anger. It empowers us to formulate anger in a productive way, allowing us the courage to see the bigger picture and to expand the level of consciousness, whereas aggression comes at the expense of all the other ideas in the room. Aggression doesn't allow for other voices to be heard, whereas assertiveness comes with a cooperative spirit.

This requires mindfulness and self-awareness. It is here, at this level of communication, where we can articulate our needs or opinions with confidence, clarity, fairness, and reason—most importantly, *so that others can hear what we're actually saying*! Assertive Communication empowers us to "source out" the root of our anger and heal it so that we don't have to be triggered over and over, unnecessarily.

The best way to explain a trigger is when someone says or does something that hits an "emotional nerve" within us—similar to touching a decayed tooth with the tine of a metal fork. It is a fear deeply embedded in our body and psyche.

The obvious solution for a trigger is to remove the source of the pain (i.e., the rotting tooth), but denial and projection prevent us from seeing this! Instead, we just try to avoid anyone or anything that may trigger the pain, making it about them rather than about healing ourselves!

Melody Beattie writes about this in *Finding Your Way Home*:

Sometimes unresolved guilt and shame—feelings we need to release and heal—get in the way of our accepting and being who our soul wants us to be. These feelings don't magically disappear. They'll come out in extraordinary ways if they're not cleared. We'll become defensive and at times say the most peculiar things. People may not be able to understand us or know what we mean. What we're really doing is defending ourselves against our own attack. Sometimes we'll project our guilt and shame—our lessons—onto another person. We'll tell people what they should or shouldn't do and what they're doing wrong. If we listen carefully to what we're saying, we'll discover we're really talking to and about ourselves.

Think of it this way: each of us has grown up believing certain personality traits are the most unacceptable, unlovable, undesirable, and unwanted. Most likely, we (or someone close to us—a parent or sibling) were shamed for behaving this same way at some point. When we stumble upon someone who behaves with these unacceptable, unlovable, undesirable, and unwanted qualities, we feel triggered. Instead of realizing they have triggered a belief in us, we reject the person. Psychologists call this "projection"—a brilliant defense mechanism of the brain.

Sigmund Freud's daughter, Anna, first introduced the concept of projection in 1937 as a survival skill by which desires we cannot accept as our own are placed in the outside world and attributed to someone else: *It's not me. It's you!*

Iyanla Vanzant describes it this way in her book *In the Meantime*:

> Sooner or later, we must all accept the fact that in a relationship the only person you are dealing with is yourself. Your partner does no more than reveal your stuff to you. Your fear! Your anger! Your pattern! Your craziness! As long as you insist on pointing the finger out there, at them, you will continue to miss out on the divine opportunity to clear out your stuff. Here is a meantime tip: we love in others what we love in ourselves. We despise in others what we cannot see in ourselves!

The concept of projection made me question every unpleasant or failed relationship I've ever had. Looking back, was it the other person's fault or could it have been me and I didn't see it? Could I have been projecting my unfinished business?

*Of course, I could have been!*

When someone can evoke extreme emotions within us—no

matter if it's our child, our parent, our partner, or a stranger on the street—we must realize it is *never* about them (nor is the way *other* people act about *us*). They may have been thoughtless or cruel. That's their stuff. Our reaction, on the other hand, is entirely ours.

A defensive or aggressive reaction occurs because they have triggered a neuro-association to past pain—a feeling we'd do anything to avoid, even if it means sabotaging ourselves. Wounded people get triggered and triggered people wound. And don't kid yourself: we are all wounded in some way!

The next time you feel yourself being triggered, getting ready to react aggressively, try this process described below instead . . . You'll need a journal to write out your responses to questions 1 through 9.

### Releasing Your Triggers

1. Who is triggering me? (Write down his or her name.) What behavior is triggering me? (Be very clear about the behavior. Write it down. Feel free to refer back to the different Emotional Sub-Archetypes as examples of personalities that trigger you.)
2. How does it make me feel when I'm around someone who is acting this way?
3. Who acted this way when I was growing up? Who taught me that this way of behaving is unacceptable and inappropriate?
4. When do I first remember acting this same way myself? How old was I? What was happening? (Remember as much as possible.)
5. How did it make me feel to be called _____ (the triggering behavior).

6. How have I overcompensated to not be _____ (the triggering behavior) ever again?

7. How has overcompensating hurt me? How has overcompensating actually helped me at times? (There is a lesson or gift in everything.)

8. Am I willing to accept that *all* people act out in less-than-desirable ways at times and that this behavior is simply one of these undesirable ways? If so, am I willing to forgive _____ (say the person's name from step 1) for behaving this way? If not, why not? When did *I* become so self-righteous and judgmental?

9. Am I willing to forgive the person who behaved this way while I was growing up? Can I also forgive the person who taught me to be ashamed about acting this way? Can I forgive myself for once acting this same way? Besides, who says this behavior is *so* unacceptable? (There is a gift in everything!)

10. Now, here is where the big healing takes place: Once you've identified the undesirable or unacceptable behavior, stand in front of a mirror, look into your own eyes, and say over and over, "I am _____." (Fill in the blank with the undesirable behavior.) Say it out loud until something in you shifts from shame, fear, or anger into neutrality, even acceptance. Owning an emotionally charged word takes the sting out of it. Once the sting is gone, you will be far less triggered and more at peace. And the really great part: you'll stop attracting people who embody this "unacceptable" behavior!

You may think that number 10, in particular, is counterintuitive and that it goes against all you've learned about repeating positive affirmations to retrain your brain, but I promise you: until you make peace with the most undesirable qualities and reclaim this disowned part of yourself, nothing will give you peace long term. People will always be able to rattle your chain.

> **Doing the "I am _____" exercise neutralizes your deepest fears.**
> **Very soon other people's opinions and actions won't affect you.**

I remember the first time I actually did this process myself. I was so upset and frustrated with a family member who was always acting aggressively with me. I felt he was a demanding, difficult, angry, bossy person who often behaved like a Ruler. It was his way or the highway! So, instead of fighting with him and being upset for weeks, I tried this instead:

"I am difficult and demanding. I am an angry person. I am the Ruler!"

I said it over and over and over for a good ten minutes, maybe longer! Strangely, I found myself shifting from an emotional state of extreme discomfort (I did not like repeating this out loud as I didn't feel I was a difficult, demanding, or angry person) into sorrow and fear, which continued to rise up into frustration and anger, and then, magically, as if some state of grace overtook me, I began to smile. *I got it!*

*Unconsciously*, my fear of being "found out" that I could be angry, difficult, or demanding was so huge that I projected this fear onto others and then did everything in my power to overcompensate; to prove that I, myself, did *not* own any of these "unacceptable qualities." From undermanaging my employees, letting people treat me any way they wanted, showing up late (especially at family events), or acting like a "dumb blonde" in order to appear at ease, relaxed, and certainly *not* difficult or controlling, I worked hard to ensure that others saw me as "Mother Earth"—gentle, saintly, and very relaxed. This made me happy. But the alternative was more than I could bear!

*I didn't want anyone to know that, deep down, I could be bossy, controlling, and overly protective! How embarrassing!*

The gift in embracing the Ruler rather than trying to bury her in the proverbial basement (in my unconscious mind), was my beginning to see her as a gift; she brought a level of protection and security to my life. She was my "quality control." Why should I be ashamed of her? Perhaps, she was trying to teach me that I needed more protection, security, and rules for myself?

By denying her (whether in front of others or just to myself), I was creating a serious disconnect within! The more I disowned her, the more fragmented I felt. Rather than feeling self-loving, safe, and whole, I felt more at odds with myself. Less empowered. More afraid.

Besides, the truth is I never *truly* felt like Mother Earth either! I always thought people would eventually figure out that I was flawed, selfish, and demanding. It took a lot of work, I discovered, to hide the Ruler and all of her reserved, domineering, angry, controlling ways.

Once I embraced her as the part of me that needed to protect me—to help me create rules, boundaries, and safety—the less I felt ashamed of her. *She knew* that *I knew* that she was there and that, should I need her, *I would call upon her.*

The Ruler certainly didn't need to run the show *or* be hidden away. She was a part of me, *but not me!*

This is what it means to integrate the wounded or fragmented aspects of ourselves back into the wholeness of who we are. As Jane Fonda said so eloquently on OWN's *Master*

*Class,* "You aren't meant to be perfect. You're meant to be whole."

The wonderful part was that without this shame, I stopped projecting the Ruler onto others—which meant I didn't need to keep attracting controlling, aggressive, difficult, and demanding people into my life to show me where I wasn't protecting myself! The Ruler taught me how to set stronger boundaries—in my life! She impressed upon me that no one had the right to hurt, abuse, or betray me. She was the Queen and would not stand for injustice. I could finally see things clearly. It was then that I was able to heal or release many of my unhealthy relationships.

When it came to the family member who I'd always viewed as the Ruler, I was able to see how wounded *he* was, too. I was able to see how many of *my* behaviors triggered him. I realized that deep down, he was angry because he loved me and worried about me but didn't know how to communicate his fear properly. I felt attacked when really all he wanted to do was protect me.

So I set an intention to show up differently and to not fall back into old patterns. I maintained my dignity, self-advocacy, and assertiveness when I spoke to him. I held space for the relationship to blossom. We both began treating each other with more respect. We both knew we could never go back to the old way of communicating. It was time to expand our relationship.

The exciting part was realizing it was never about him (as cruel and demanding as he'd been); it was about me and the role I'd chosen to play—the Emotional Sub-Archetype I'd developed at a very young age. I was always the Scared Child when it came to him. No wonder he acted like the angry Ruler with me!

I continue to remind myself:

"Only wounded people get triggered and only I can heal my own wounds."

The same thing applies to you: It is never about them. It is always about you. Learn from your suffering. Face it. See it. Accept it. Grow. Evolve. Expand. This is an empowering realization! It means we can heal ourselves without receiving anything from the person who hurt us!

Another way to help you discover what your hidden triggers are is to pay attention to which Emotional Sub-Archetypes bother, upset, or irritate you the most. In other words, if someone called you a Martyr, would that upset you more than being referred to as a Charmer? Would being called a Victim or a Chubby Bubby be worse than being called a Warrior or a Micromanager? What's the worst thing one can call you?

Once you can identify the archetypes that trigger you the most (the ones you'd never want to be called), you can once again do the "Release Your Triggers" exercise above. *This time realizing that it is you (and always has been you) who has been triggering you!*

> **Our shame is our own worst enemy. We will do almost anything to hide it from the world, even overcompensating— even creating the opposite Emotional Sub-Archetype for the world to see!**

Our behavior is always our responsibility. But without outlets for our frustrations, even the best person in the world can become like that beautiful bottle of champagne—agitate it too many times and it'll explode! Don't let this be you! Learn to see where you are not expressing yourself in an empowered way!

When you feel yourself "flooding," or being overwhelmed,

step away and take the time to do the "Release Your Triggers" exercise!

Now, I'm not saying people will never confuse, irritate, or upset you but you will find that your triggers become fewer and further between.

Here's something I will promise you: reading this exercise and actually doing it are two different things! Until you actually do the "Release Your Triggers" process, you cannot imagine the freedom you will find!

# CHAPTER FOUR

# Empowered Communication Begins

## "TRANSCEND"

> Your task is not to seek for love, but merely to seek
> and find all the barriers
> within yourself that you have built against it.
>
> RUMI

In this chapter, you will learn and practice the art of Empowered Communication, while ascending into the higher levels of consciousness.

You will discover how to advocate for yourself in a way that lifts up those around you, and you will discover how to listen to others without losing yourself. Ultimately, you will learn how to expand your consciousness to become the fully empowered Adult!

Let's begin with Assertive Communication . . .

# Assertive Communication

I think of Assertive Communication as the "bridge" between the lower levels of communication—Passive, Passive-Aggressive, and Aggressive—and the higher levels—Acceptance, Love, Joy, and Peace.

When your communication falls into the lower levels, you are acting on the defensive or the offensive. You certainly aren't neutral. You have an agenda. You're in a power struggle. You're angry! Or worse—you're sad and scared and you're not sure how to advocate for yourself. You're unable to put your best face forward because you're working so hard to protect yourself.

As you learn how to practice Assertive Communication, though, you will begin to navigate your life in a more emboldened way. Things actually begin to get easier as you let up on that fierce grip and become your authentic self! It is here that the Adult Archetype is first witnessed.

But let's be honest: when anger erupts, it's challenging at times to channel it into assertiveness—a safe, neutral zone. Aggressiveness, on the other hand, may temporarily feel more domineering or powerful, but its consequences are painful in the long term, which is why we must learn the art of Empowered Communication.

Initially, anger can feel like a jolt of adrenaline, almost like putting your hand on a hot burner. Revved up, anger stimulates our senses. For many people, this is the most powerful they *ever* feel. Anger can be addictive—physically and emotionally!

The great news is that "anger is jet fuel," and when employed properly, we can use it to soar in our lives. When abused, anger will ruin lives—including our own.

Empowered people know that anger is a natural and often legitimate emotion, and they have learned that, when misdirected, it destroys. It limits and constricts our lives—our health, wealth, love, energy, passion, and vitality. The Adult Archetype knows that long-term needs outweigh immediate needs, unless there is obvious imminent danger. We have to learn how to hit the Pause button and think before we speak.

Once we realize we can express ourselves in an honest way, without the intent to hurt others and without allowing others to hurt us, we are on our way toward operating as empowered women or men! This is what Assertive Communication looks and feels like. It is the first massive shift from the lower levels of consciousness to the higher.

## THE ESSENCE OF ASSERTIVE COMMUNICATION

Assertive Communication means having the courage to look at yourself and at the bigger picture, and articulate your needs with clarity, confidence, and composure. Most important, you are communicating in a way that allows others actually to hear what you're saying. This takes self-awareness, insight, and reason. You must be able to both speak *and* listen effectively.

Assertive Communication feels much the same as releasing that submerged beach ball: relief! Instead of suppressing your feelings, you are allowing and communicating them in a "win-win" way. All it requires is letting go of that fierce grip—the fear that your needs don't matter or won't be acknowledged. This requires trust. It's amazing how people respond to this communication style and strategy!

The truth is that many of us (especially women) want to skip this level. We don't want to acknowledge or deal with our "uncomfortable" or "unhappy" feelings. But if we try to dodge this step by avoiding a conversation that needs to be had, and instead we simply try to move higher into Accepting Communication, we'll discover ourselves eventually being pulled back down into anger again. Remember, whatever is repressed will find a way to be expressed. You can't avoid your needs in hopes of becoming an accepting person. The secret is speaking calmly, clearly, and truthfully—it's where authentic power *begins* to blossom. It is the root of all empowerment.

Assertiveness acknowledges *our* self-worth and dignity as well as that of other people—no matter who they are and no matter what they've done.

As challenging as this initially may be, once this level is mastered it becomes much easier to stand up for your beliefs and/or yourself, while still communicating with respectful words and intentions.

Once you embrace this level, your life begins to unfold with ease and certainty. You'll realize there is nothing you can't handle. Nothing you can't address and deal with. It's all about the way you communicate! You don't need to worry about having a confrontation once you embrace Empowered Communication!

Empowered people—both men and women—have learned to manage their emotions without repressing them and without allowing them to oppress others. They're doing the work to heal their own wounds and triggers. Their intentions are to speak their truth with dignity and respect (energy follows intention). They know their life matters. They have a healthy sense of their rights as well as the rights of others. They aim for cooperation and collaboration and a "win-win" approach!

When an assertive person interacts with another human being, his or her intention is to make the situation a "win-win" for everyone, which might involve compromise and negotiation but which leaves both parties feeling as though their voices were heard and acknowledged. This approach is the key difference that distinguishes assertiveness from both aggression and passivity. It is higher resonating, and it requires us to pay attention to context.

Context is what allows us to know the most appropriate response. In other words, as you climb the Empowerment Spectrum you will view the same situation differently—from a higher perspective—than you did several levels lower. It's not so up close and personal. You begin to realize it's not all about you, or not even necessarily what you thought it was about. As context expands, so does meaning. You see that there are other variables happening.

This is why I stress to my children and my clients never to make life-changing decisions when they feel passive, passive-aggressive, or aggressive. Don't make major changes when you're feeling disempowered. You don't have a clear enough perspective at these levels: *Sometimes you have to sleep on it! Sometimes you just need to have a good cry! Sometimes you need to talk it out first!*

It takes courage to look within rather than pointing the finger outward. It takes courage to not settle for less than you need while still listening to what those around you are saying. It takes courage to be an Assertive Communicator.

Nathaniel Branden, PhD, who is a pioneer in the field of self-esteem and self-assertiveness, writes:

> The first and basic act of self-assertion is the assertion of consciousness. This entails the choice to see, to think, to be aware, to send the light of consciousness outward toward the world and inward toward our own being. To ask questions is an act of self-assertion. To challenge authority is an act of self-assertion. To think for oneself—and

to stand by what one thinks—is the root of self-assertion. To default on this responsibility is to default on the self at the most basic level.

Note: Self-assertiveness should not be confused with mindless rebelliousness. "Self-assertiveness without consciousness is not self-assertiveness; it is drunk-driving."

We are all born with a sense of assertiveness or confidence! There was a time you felt "the truth"—you knew right from wrong. You knew what you liked or didn't like. You knew your Self! You knew you mattered!

Just look at any three-year-old. She knows exactly what she wants, what she likes, and how she feels. She is not ashamed or afraid to ask for what she wants. She feels her feelings, responds in the moment, and shakes off the rest. She trusts life. She trusts herself. She trusts you.

Yet somewhere along the way, most of us were taught to feel scared, limited, unsafe, and imperfect. By the time we (previously) joyful children became adults, we learned to be distrustful, disconnected, and ready to give up on our dreams and ambitions.

Most of us need to relearn the truth we already knew as young kids: life is unlimited, abundant, and safe. Not to mention, it's our birthright to enjoy it!

But this takes "waking up" and recontextualizing things so that we can regain our childlike innocence, happiness, and belief in life and in ourselves again. This takes mindfulness! Self-awareness! Courage!

Mindfulness is far different from concentration. "It is a discipline whereby you maintain clear moment-to-moment awareness of what is happening internally and externally, rather than coloring your interpretation with your emotions or being engaged 'elsewhere,' deep in thought." This is an important skill to think about in the context of your communication style. By seeing things through neutral, impartial lenses you are better able to remain empowered. You retain some distance from the situation at hand, a form of healthy detachment that allows you to stay calm and logical. Nonattachment can sound like a cold, stern, indifferent emotion, but it is actually a very loving position. Remaining nonattached means being open to what is—doing all that you can do within reasonable means, then allowing the nature of things to unfold. Again, this takes mindfulness.

Ellen J. Langer, PhD, is a professor of psychology at Harvard University. Her brilliant book *Mindfulness* points out that many "outcome-oriented people" often live their lives in search of achievement rather than experiencing "the process," which causes mindlessness.

> From kindergarten on, the focus of schooling is usually on goals rather than on the process by which they are achieved. This single-minded pursuit of one outcome or another, from tying shoelaces to getting into Harvard, makes it difficult to have a mindful attitude about life.

Too many people are mindlessly going about their lives, living in a reactionary state and striving for a specific goal, rather than consciously, mindfully remaining in a state of present awareness. They've stopped paying attention. They've stopped feeling. They're multitasking to the point of absent-mindedness, constantly pulled into drama and dysfunction by their external experiences. They never shift beyond Passive, Passive-Aggressive, and Aggressive Communication.

Assertiveness is an art in and of itself. It requires us to be mindful, aware, and courageous; to wake up and be present, to expand our level of consciousness by paying attention to the "now"—the present moment—with all of our senses. It requires us to know, *for certain*, that our life matters, our needs matter, and our happiness matters.

For years I've used a simple acronym—WOMAN—as my Assertiveness Cue. This acronym works perfectly for men, too:

- **W**hat are my intentions?
- **O**verlook the obvious
- **M**anage my emotions
- **A**sk the right questions
- **N**egotiate new healthy boundaries

## The WOMAN Acronym

As I've already pointed out, being assertive is necessary to being empowered. Being present and open to different perspectives are important aspects of assertiveness. If we cling to our point of view, we become unable to grow, evolve, and expand.

Let's look now at the WOMAN acronym:

### *WHAT* ARE MY INTENTIONS?

Intention is the origin of outcome. Energy follows intention. These are the cause and the effect: intention is the cause, and outcome is the effect. By learning to be mindful of our intentions, we instantly create a clear direction for ourselves. Our intentions have a surprisingly persuasive way of transforming our lives and our relationships. The best way to imagine this is to consider that what we think about directly influences our reality.

For example, setting the intention for peace will automatically incline you toward a more Peaceful Communication style. On the other hand, an intention to be right will lead you toward aggression. When you aren't clear on your intentions, you will find yourself pulled in different directions without any sense of healthy boundaries.

Just imagine if, before every encounter (especially normally stressful situations), you were to ask yourself: "What are my intentions?" or "What do I want to happen?" or "What archetype do I want to be in?" or, my favorite, "If I could wave a magic wand and I was guaranteed success, what would I wish for?"

Some other sample questions might look like these:

- What do I feel? What do I want to feel instead?
- What would an empowered woman (or man) do in this same situation?
- What would courage have me do? And am I willing to do it?

When you go into a situation knowing what you want, you are in a much stronger position to advocate for yourself. This leads us to the next step in the WOMAN acronym . . .

### *OVERLOOK* THE OBVIOUS

We all get caught up in the moment, pulled into what I call the obvious—receiving the mean letter, hearing the cruel words, rebuking the hostile coworker, confronting the passive-aggressive in-law, inflicting the road rage, or getting entangled in whatever the drama or chaos of the moment seems to be. But if we want to be empowered, we must learn to Overlook the Obvious and remain mindful of our intentions and aware of the truth.

We must rise above the situation and not get pulled into the proverbial "forest," where we can see only the trees. We must practice stopping ourselves from sweating the small stuff. Stop getting pulled into drama and dysfunction. Look beyond the obvious distractions so that we can focus on the real steps that we must take to achieve our intentions.

Think about a judge in a courtroom. One of the crucial qualities required in the judicial system is neutrality, or nonattachment, whereby a judge can be impartial about his or her decision-making process. Judges must be reasonable, looking only at the evidence rather than the emotions, weighing things out objectively. We call this taking the thirty-thousand-foot view. This is what we, too, must learn to do! Don't get caught up in the details.

Spiritual teacher Byron Katie has a process she calls "The Work," in which she encourages us to ask these four questions whenever we find ourselves getting pulled into drama and suffering:

1. Is it true? (Yes or no. If no, move to 3.)
2. Can you absolutely know that it's true? (Yes or no.)
3. How do you react when you believe that thought?
4. Who would you be without the thought?

If we can move beyond our self-righteousness and pride, we can learn to overlook the obvious and stay in an empowered place. As Rob Bell shares so succinctly in his book *Sex God*: "*This* is rarely about *this*. *This* is usually about *that*." The secret is figuring out what "that" really is and responding authentically.

Once things have calmed down, you can try to read between the lines, and look objectively at both perspectives. Being able to pause, count to ten, think about how you feel and what you want to feel instead—*your intentions*—and then react appropriately—these skills take self-awareness.

> It takes a deep desire to want to know "the truth," without agenda. This is how you know that you are evolving from the lower levels of communication into the higher ones!

As a mother, I often employ this technique to understand why my children behave certain ways, without taking it personally. For instance, when my two-year-old was having a temper tantrum, I would step outside of my own feelings to take into account the time of day, if she was hungry, how much sleep she had the night before, whether she was overtired, what was happening in her outer world (e.g., sibling rivalry), how her dad and I were getting along, and so forth. The more I did this, the easier it was to find the patterns in my daughter's behavior. I was able to overlook her tantrum and find the real trigger behind her actions.

If I let myself get pulled into my child's flip out, I would be reacting at her emotional level rather than observing her objectively to understand what was at the root of her unhappiness. I would be the Child Archetype parenting a child.

I believe I've always been able to stay fairly calm with my kids because I resonated in acceptance and love rather than guilt and fear. I parented from the Adult Archetype.

You must apply this same wisdom and neutrality to all your encounters, which also means examining and discarding personal beliefs that aren't serving you, particularly when you realize they are opinions rather than facts. If you have to assert yourself (and this is very different from defend yourself), you will with courage and composure. You will not get caught up in the details or the "he said, she said." Once you've learned to overlook the obvious to begin to manage other people's responses, you will have an easier time managing your own responses to even a difficult situation.

## *MANAGE* MY EMOTIONS

One of the things that is so spectacular about human beings is how our bodies have their own "truth barometer," almost like an internal GPS (global positioning system) guiding us:

Red light: *Stop!*
Yellow light: *Proceed with caution!*
Green light: *Go!*

This internal compass continually points us toward our true Self, and away from things that will take us out of alignment. When we allow ourselves to "feel our feelings" rather than numb, deny, or escape them, we can access our inner GPS easily and effortlessly.

For years I've taught my clients the difference between a feeling and an emotion. A feeling is simply a visceral reaction to an outside stimulus. It has no thought. It has no *judgment*. It is not right or wrong. It simply is, happening here and now. It has no attachment or connection to the past or future. It isn't angry, sad, or happy; it just *is*—a sign, an instantaneous sensation within your body—*it is your "gut instinct."* For example: This is causing me discomfort . . . This gives me relief . . . This feels expansive . . . This feels constrictive . . . A feeling moves quickly and doesn't linger. Feeling your feelings is mandatory if you want to be empowered!

The secret is learning how to feel a feeling without becoming it.

*Emotions are different from feelings.* Emotions have the added component of thought. When we react to a feeling we begin telling ourselves a story about it; we attach a belief to it.

As you know already, our beliefs are created by our view of the world, driven by our Emotional Sub-Archetype or life script. Beliefs create emotions. Emotions create chemical reactions within the body—almost instantaneously. Chemicals are addictive.

Often an interaction can begin to break down when people allow their emotions into the driver's seat. Before you know it, your "gut instinct"—a simple feeling designed to move you in the right direction—has turned into an uncomfortable exchange triggered by your emotional baggage and self-limiting beliefs. The healthier you are (meaning you've healed your triggers), the easier managing your emotions will be.

Practice checking in with your internal GPS throughout the day by asking yourself, "What do I feel right now?" Be an observer of your emotions rather than a judge. Witness them without reacting. Feel your feelings without trying to numb or solve them. And remember, "This too shall pass."

By remaining mindful of your intentions, without getting dragged into the drama (and this often means overlooking the obvious), you can learn to "feel a feeling" without overreacting to it. In other words, you'll go with the flow but not because of it. This way, you will be able to keep your intentions at the forefront of your actions and not fall into the trap of giving your power away.

## ASK THE RIGHT QUESTIONS

As you're evaluating a situation, be it a negotiation at work or a heated conversation with a family member, you must ask yourself questions that will expand your consciousness and lift your emotions toward peace. You mustn't ask yourself questions that will force you down toward passivity or shame.

Asking yourself the right questions will allow you quickly to ascend into a higher perspective, which will lead you toward freedom, liberation, and personal empowerment. Remember, scientists have told us that passive people ask disempowered questions, while empowered people ask empowered questions!

*This is a sample list of questions that you could ask yourself (in sequence) on your way to becoming the Adult Archetype:*

1. Shame: What happened that made me feel so worthless and ashamed?
2. Guilt: Why do *I* feel so badly? What did *I* do (or what didn't I do) that I wish I could change?
3. Apathy: Deep down, whom do I ultimately blame for this? (Hint: Tell yourself the truth!)
4. Grief: How did their actions hurt me, change me, or keep me stuck?
5. Fear: What fears are stopping me from moving forward? (Hint: Fear of telling the truth, being alone, failing, shining too brightly, etc.)
6. Desire: If I wasn't afraid, I would _____. (Fill in the blank with your deepest desires.)
7. Anger: Is this situation unacceptable, unfair, and/or unhealthy?
8. Pride: How can I be so certain?
9. Courage: What would courage have me do?
10. Willingness: Am I willing to do it?

Courage is the magic place, resonating at a level of energy powerful enough to shift you into Empowered Communication. It is here where you must take the final, crucial step in our WOMAN acronym . . .

## *NEGOTIATE* NEW HEALTHY BOUNDARIES

I've saved the toughest one for last: Healthy boundaries create healthy relationships. Unhealthy boundaries create unhealthy relationships. This is what we mean by "we teach people how to treat us by the way we treat ourselves."

Without healthy boundaries, others can touch us how they want, treat us how they want, and do whatever they wish with our possessions. Most often, by the time we're upset, we've allowed someone to overstep our boundaries. But let's be honest: setting boundaries takes courage, confidence, and assertiveness!

By establishing clear boundaries, we define ourselves in relation to others—including with our own family! To do this, we must be able to identify, honor, and respect our own worth and recognize the unacceptable behavior that someone else is imposing on us. Otherwise, it would be like keeping the front door of your home unlocked and open all night, allowing strangers and criminals to come inside and steal from you. You have the right to say no (and yes), to feel safe, and to decide whom you will let in, and how much you will allow—and this includes with your partner, friends, mother, father, children, family members, siblings, neighbors, and business associates! The trouble is, when we don't know our own worth, we struggle as adults with setting healthy boundaries.

Just the other day, I was speaking to a beautiful, smart, talented woman who was experiencing extreme anxiety. When we talked further, she said her boss had been coming on to her, but she didn't want to hurt his feelings or make him feel rejected by putting her foot down. She allowed him to get too close, to say inappropriate things, and to grope her. She hated how she felt around him, but she didn't know how to establish a healthy boundary. How could she say something now when she'd let it go on for this long? She felt somehow to blame!

*(This is all part of the grooming process most women have experienced from the time they were young!)*

Besides, she knew, deep down, that he was a "good man," she said. He was married, had a wonderful wife and many grandchildren. He was even the deacon at their local church!

I gently explained that most of us didn't witness healthy boundary setting while we were growing up. We weren't taught how to say no. Our parents were either too rigid or too porous—meaning overly protective of us or not protective enough—teaching us to be afraid, unable, or unsure of how to protect ourselves. We were groomed for shame, guilt, and secrets. And now, as adults, we still don't know how to assert ourselves in empowered, impartial, healthy ways.

In my life, it seemed to me that no one in my family seemed to care if I was dead or alive. The message I received was that I was on my own. As much as I wanted to protect myself, I didn't know how. I didn't have the tools. I was still a child myself. No one "modeled" it to me. Maybe no one had taught them Empowered Communication either?

In any case, no wonder my life was a series of catastrophic events. I had a blind spot when it came to protecting myself. I could take care of and empower everyone else—especially other women—but I somehow seemed to drop the ball when it came to me.

This is why, when dealing with triggers, you need to be very clear about the behaviors that you find to be upsetting or frustrating. Once you've healed your own stuff, you'll know whether something is a trigger versus an inappropriate behavior: "Has he or she crossed a boundary or am I being overly sensitive?"

Learning to set healthy boundaries can feel uncomfortable, even scary, because for most of us it's foreign, especially if our parents or caretakers didn't protect us properly. As adults, we struggle with low self-esteem and little self-worth.

What if we say no and others get mad at us? What if they leave us? What if they hate us? Abandon us? Betray us? Judge us? Hurt us? Gossip about us? Try to destroy our lives for telling the truth?

*Yes—this is courageous work!*

> **Never let a bully stop you from being your own empowered, assertive person! No one has that right!**

The sad part is that we often unknowingly continue to give off the vibe that it's okay to treat us in an inappropriate way. We've become either the Child Archetype, who oversteps and overtakes, or the Parent Archetype, who gives too much and allows too much. Sometimes, we just swing back and forth between the two. In any case, codependent, unhealthy relationships ensue when we don't have healthy boundaries!

If you feel that someone has crossed a boundary, it is not only okay, it is *necessary* that you arrange a time to chat with this person. Honest, courageous conversation is required if you want to be an empowered adult.

*Set your intentions for the desired outcome and then follow this simple, four-step formula for healthy boundary setting:*

1. When you _____. (Fill in the blank with the behavior that is making you uncomfortable.)
2. I feel _____. (State your emotion without overdramatizing.)
3. Would you be willing to _____? (Ask for what you need instead.)
4. If you can't do this for me, I will _____. (State your consequence.)

Step 4 is the hardest part, but describing what you will do to protect the boundary you've set is crucial. It is then equally important that you follow through with the consequence. And be sure "the time fits the crime." Don't set yourself, and the other person, up for a ridiculous punishment that neither of you is able to maintain.

Boundary setting is not about trying to manipulate or control another person; you can be responsible for only your part. This is about becoming an Assertive Communicator.

If other people are angry that you are trying to negotiate with them, you can't take on their emotions. This is where a little mental "cord cutting" may have to take place. For me, this is the hardest part of boundary setting. They are responsible for themselves, and you must overlook their obvious dislike of what you are trying to do. You are creating a healthier and more empowered life for yourself, and you are actually teaching them healthy behavior. Besides, maybe you setting and maintaining a healthy boundary is exactly the medicine they need.

If you are new to boundary setting, expect the people in your life to test you! No one likes the rules to change, especially if there have been few to no rules in the past. You can even expect your own disempowered Emotional Sub-Archetype(s) to test you, that is, you may experience a battle within! These aspects of ourselves struggle with healthy boundary setting: they are either too porous or too rigid.

Speaking of too rigid, don't become so inflexible in your boundaries that you self-righteously demand, snub, demean, or exclude people if you feel they have overstepped you. If you remain calm, clear, and fair about your intentions, you will teach the people in your life healthy, empowered behavior. And that is great news for everyone!

The important thing to keep in mind is that healthy boundary setting isn't just so you can teach the people in your life how to treat you, it also requires that you understand how to treat others. In this day and age, with Facebook, Twitter, e-mail, texting—you name it—we have this false idea that we have the right to get ahold of whomever we want, whenever we want, and that they should reply to us promptly!

Just because the world is at our fingertips doesn't mean we have permission to poke at people anytime of the day or night. This also applies to our professional relationships. Be cognizant of the time of day or the day of the week that you send messages to others. If it is late at night or on a weekend, be sure to explain that you are working but that you do not expect them to reply until they are able to do so.

All people have the right to privacy, space, and the time they need to make decisions. We can't force ourselves on anyone and demand that we get answers when we want them.

Once we've reached this point, we are really learning to trust ourselves again; we may even be feeling some of that childlike love, excitement, and creativity. When this happens, we feel ourselves shift into a higher level of communication called Acceptance.

## Accepting Communication and Beyond

Accepting Communication is where all the good stuff starts manifesting easily. We've crossed over the bridge of Assertive Communication, and we're standing on higher ground. We're showing up in the world as an empowered Adult. We've surrendered our fear—examined it, learned from it, and expanded it—in order to become powerful.

For many people the concept of surrendering means giving up, waving the white flag, admitting defeat. This is the opposite of what I'm suggesting. Surrendering is seeking truth over seeking compliance. It is not knowing and yet, completely knowing that all is okay. It is the realization that what you defend against, you create. The more you dig your heels in, the more resistance you'll experience.

The empowered choice is to do all that you possibly can to expand the situation to its highest place and then let go. See what unfolds. Trust in the signs without judgment. You "let it be," just as the Beatles said to do.

Being an Accepting Communicator doesn't mean you accept bad or inappropriate treatment; instead, it means you are wise enough to see that you can't change anything until you first accept that it is what it is. It also allows you to weigh things out and to see if it is even within your control or your circumstance to change. Besides, you know now how to set a healthy boundary, should you find yourself feeling frustrated or taken advantage of.

Accepting Communication allows you to become open-minded, calm, and reasonable. You relax and trust. You live and let live.

> God, grant me the serenity to
> accept the things I cannot change,
> The courage to change the things I can;
> and the wisdom to know the difference.
> REINHOLD NIEBUHR

Accepting Communication impresses upon us that life is simply a series of causes and effects. Being upset at the aftermath (as maddening or unacceptable as it may be) will waste our energy because there are so many variables that led us to where we are today.

Yes—we must acknowledge and understand our past in order to make better decisions today, but focusing on what was will not change what will come. Things happened that we didn't understand, didn't want, and didn't like. But when we resonate in Accepting Communication, we accept that although we can't see the bigger picture, it doesn't mean there isn't one. Instead of being self-righteous or "absolutely certain," we evaluate our results and look for discrepancies or consistencies in our patterns; this will empower us to expand our possibilities rather than contract into them. This is how acceptance is achieved.

The Adult Archetype understands that when something triggers or upsets them, it is because of a fear they have bought into—a pattern that must be healed. They breathe into their resistance and ask:

> When did I learn that what is happening is wrong? When did I learn that this person or experience is wrong? When did I learn that feeling this way is wrong? From whom did I learn this? Can I learn from and accept this instead of reject and resist it? What if this is how it is supposed to be?

As I've already mentioned, we were *all* taught that certain ways of acting, feeling, or being are wrong, unacceptable, or undesirable. We've been taught to be judgmental and self-righteous—especially with ourselves. We were taught to reject certain qualities and attributes. We were taught to lie and reject liars. We were taught to rebuke, censure, and reprimand those who are different from us. We were taught that the only way to be empowered was to stand up for what we believe in and hold our ground . . . even if we're not 100 percent sure!

Until you accept that you were taught a whole slew of contradictory beliefs, mostly about judging, evaluating, and criticizing, you will not be able to love and accept anyone fully—*especially yourself!* You'll live your life waiting for the approval of others. This will rob you of your power. You'll make choices searching for "their acceptance" rather than living true to your own ambition.

Ambition is not a word to fear. It is simply the get-up-and-go to move in the direction of your passion and purpose. When you focus on your ambitions rather than the need to be approved of, you ascend into your authentic Self much more easily!

*Here are some examples of questions to help you be mindful of your level of acceptance:*

1. Do I accept myself even when others don't?
2. Do I accept my body and self-image—today—as I am?
3. Do I accept that I may fail?
4. Do I accept that we won't all see things the same way and that that's okay?
5. Do I accept others without accepting their behavior?
6. Do I accept that others may not agree with my desires or decisions?
7. Do I accept that I may not agree with the desires or decisions of others?
8. Do I accept our differences?

Whenever you feel yourself becoming controlling, fearful, or aggressive, ask yourself: "If I were more accepting with less self-righteousness and pride, what would I surrender?"

I used to confuse love and acceptance with codependence and enabling. I couldn't figure out how to accept someone without accepting his or her unhealthy behavior. After attending a few Al-Anon meetings and devouring all of Melody Beattie's books, I realized that *love holds space*. This term means that love allows you to speak your truth, and then it believes the truth will blossom; it waits patiently, while continuing to hold and expand the space for your loved one to meet you.

And yes, sometimes we may have to "hold space" from a distance. This is called tough love. And it is *so* tough sometimes . . .

I know stepping away from a relationship (even a bad one) feels sad, even scary. The best way I've coached someone through a difficult breakup (and this may mean ending a relationship or taking a time-out with a friend, family member, lover, spouse, boss, or employee) is by reminding him or her that the door is not necessarily shut permanently. He or she is simply setting a healthy boundary, for now.

Here's the truth: love always finds a way. If it is meant to be, the relationship will matter too much for both of you to let it go completely. Maybe a little space and perspective is exactly what is needed. Don't panic. Allow it to unfold. Accept what is. Don't force it. Trust in the power of love.

It reminds me of a cute line in the movie *The Best Exotic Marigold Hotel*:

> In India, we have a saying: "In the end, it will all be okay. If it is not okay, it is not the end."

However, in the meantime, space may be exactly what is required. Just be sure you aren't "checking out" and emotionally neglecting or dismissing someone you care for. Remember, careless disregard is the same as intentionally hurting someone.

## "LETTING GO" VERSUS "CHECKING OUT"

After coaching thousands of people over the past twenty years, I've witnessed many people "check out" on their most important relationships and then use the enlightened line: "I'm just setting a healthy boundary. I'm letting go."

Whenever a conversation or situation gets uncomfortable, they aren't willing to dig in, listen, talk it out, look at both sides, and stay committed to finding resolution and peace. They aren't invested enough. They don't know the art of Empowered Communication. They emotionally shut down and shut off. This is called stonewalling:

> Conversation ended! Now! Who cares what you need to say? I'm done! I'm cutting you off! Over and out.

Some people stonewall their loved ones for a few hours; some do it for years! If people you care about have checked out on you, do *not* take it personally. When people check out on us, it is an example of emotional inadequacy—their inability to cope and communicate effectively. If they knew better, they'd do better, but they can't, *yet*.

If the relationship matters to you, you might say something to them such as:

> I love you. That's never going to change. But I feel sad and hurt when you ignore me. Can we talk about this? I miss you. I want you in my life. I want both of our needs to be met.

Every relationship is a negotiation. Every. Single. One.

The secret to maintaining your Emotional Edge is to catch yourself when you feel as though you're sliding down from this empowered place—in other words, before you "take the walk" over the bridge down into Aggressive Communication.

The best way to do this is to activate your WOMAN acronym. Ask yourself: "What are my intentions? Can I overlook the obvious and not get caught up in the 'he said, she said'? Will I manage my emotions and speak with dignity, honesty, and respect? What questions could I ask to expand or improve this situation rather than contract and dismantle it? And if needed, will I negotiate new healthy boundaries to teach the people in my life how to treat me?"

You can't force someone up the Empowerment Spectrum with you. You can't force someone to love you or to listen to you! You can't make someone have a healthy, empowered relationship with you, especially if they are unhealthy themselves!

Here's what you must remind yourself: learning via suffering no longer serves you. You don't have to suffer. It's a choice. What will you accept? What will you *not* accept?

*Can you accept a person and not accept a behavior?*

The answer is yes—if *you* are resonating in acceptance and love. For me, this singular step has been the most important thing I've learned in maintaining a healthy, harmonious, empowered relationship—with anyone.

Before her sad and untimely death, my friend Debbie Ford helped me through a painful breakup by asking me three important questions late one evening when we were chatting on the telephone:

1. Do you love him? My answer: *Yes.*
2. Do you trust him? My answer: *No.*

**3.** Do you respect yourself with him? My answer (after a long pause): *No, I don't . . .*

"Then, you can't be with him!" she told me, "No matter how much you love him, you don't trust him. And even worse, you don't respect yourself with him!"

I ended the relationship within a few days of that conversation—not because she told me to *but because I knew*: If nothing changed, nothing would change. I'd caught him cheating one too many times. I knew I loved him, but I couldn't accept the behavior. There was no reason for it. We had a passionate sex life.

At the time, I honestly believed I was creating space for *him* to get the help *he* needed. I was certain we'd be back together within a few months; *he'd* come around. *He'd* grow up.

Our parting was done with kindness and dignity. There was no name-calling or demonizing each other. I loved him; I just couldn't accept some of his behaviors.

I realize now that I was actually creating space *for me* to find my Self again—to chip away the clay I had layered on. I had changes to make if I was ever going to be the woman I needed to be when it came to creating and sustaining a healthy love life for myself.

I had this tendency to lose myself in relationships by becoming the primary giver (very masculine) and overloving my man to the point that I enabled him by disabling him. So afraid I wasn't worthy enough, I would do everything possible to prove I was a "good catch." I would start out in my Woman Energy but inevitably I'd fall into Mother Energy. All that proving became exhausting. Why did it surprise me when I caught him cheating, *again*? He was the naughty little boy, and I was the angry, overworked mother! It was time to cut the cord. I'd been more concerned with helping him heal his "stuff" than I was with my own.

Letting go was one of the hardest things I've ever done, but in the end, it was the right thing for me. I had so much cleaning up to do myself. I had so many "amends" to make to my own heart. The truth is, as much as I "loved" him, from day one I had been compromising myself to be with him. How could it ever have blossomed based on my losing myself to make it work?

Maybe if I had had the communication skills and empowerment that I have now the relationship could have turned out totally differently. Maybe we were soul mates. Maybe we were never meant to go on more than a few dates. Who knows? It was what it was. We did what we did. I am not angry with him anymore. I played an equal part in the dynamics; I created my reality, whether I felt victimized or not. I'd learned helplessness when it came to men. He mirrored back to me exactly what I believed!

The good news is that I now have a wonderful man who holds me in the highest regard—because I do . . . and because he respects himself just as much.

In honesty, it took me nearly five years to heal my heart enough so that I could fully receive my husband's pure and unconditional love. I had to expand my Emotional Edges. I'd been living in constrictive, fearful energy for too long—especially when it came to men. I had to learn how to trust again. That meant first learning to trust myself that I would always take care of me, and then the huge process of learning to trust others. My beliefs had to be challenged. I had to retrain my brain to see things and people through higher resonating lenses.

The first few years of my marriage were not peaches and

cream! I had to learn how to accept our differences. We both had a lot of compromising and negotiating to figure out, and we sometimes raged back and forth between the Child Archetype and the Parent Archetype. But we knew our love was strong, so we committed ourselves to finding *acceptance* with each other . . . and with ourselves! We both committed to becoming the Adult! It's still a journey at times, but one that I am so happy to be on!

Long-term relationships aren't about being the same. They are about loving each other so much you're willing to hold space for the other. It reminds me of the beautiful lyrics in the Faith Hill song: "I'll wait for you / Should I fall behind wait for me." Acceptance, reason, and love allow you to navigate during these tougher times.

(We will talk more about our intimate relationships in Chapter Seven.)

Here is something else to keep in mind: it's easy to believe you are resonating in Accepting Communication when you live alone, have few *real* friends (social media friends don't count), aren't in a serious intimate relationship, or regularly limit your time with extended family members. You may think you are at ease, but look closer: Have you simply "checked out" on yourself and your loved ones? Be sure to reflect on this. There's a fine line between having a small but strong group of trusted allies and becoming the Lone Wolf, an example archetype of someone who has "checked out."

You were designed to love and be loved, and you can do that only by giving and receiving love from other human beings. We aren't meant to be lone wolves. We're pack animals. We need each other—up close and personal.

I've seen the power that our most intimate relationships (or lack thereof) can have on our lives. When we aren't in a good place in our relationships—especially in our love life—being in a good place in the rest of our lives is much more challenging. Our relationships matter exponentially!

With that being said, if you are in an abusive, unhealthy, unfaithful, or unkind relationship, you must rise above it to regain perspective. This may mean you have to step away, *sometimes permanently*.

By taking the thirty-thousand-foot view you will discover that on some level you overlooked the signs or you somehow told yourself that unhealthy behavior was acceptable. Perhaps no one taught you how to set healthy boundaries or no one showed you how worthy and deserving you are of respect, care, and kindness; maybe you learned helplessness, and didn't realize your situation is escapable!

Looking back to the beginning of my own unhealthy relationship, there were things about the situation that didn't resonate with my personal values or sensibilities, but I chose to ignore them. I saw the signs! He wasn't fooling me. I was fooling myself, certain that I could change him to be what I wanted him to be.

My guess is that if you take a look at your circumstances, you will find at the root an experience that triggered you to operate in a wounded archetype. A power struggle ensued. You, or perhaps both of you, are losing out.

We've all heard this saying: "We teach people how to treat us by the way we treat ourselves." Do you see how, somewhere along the way, you began accepting treatment you weren't comfortable with?

> Here's the bottom line:
> You can't have love without acceptance. Besides, you can't change anything until you accept it.

Imagine the next time a loved one does something you normally find to be frustrating: instead of reacting, whisper in your head, "I accept you. I may not understand you (or agree with you) but I accept you."

Once you can accept a person or a situation, you can let go of your judgment and self-righteousness about who *you* believe he or she needs to be in order for you to approve or in order for him or her to be worthy of love. You'll express your feelings without worrying about the outcome because you trust yourself more. You will be able to negotiate your way through any conflict without being distracted by old "stories," disempowered emotions, limiting beliefs, or unfinished business—the baggage—you are bringing to the situation.

Now, this is not the same thing as allowing people to do whatever they like or to treat you inappropriately. If you simply cannot accept a behavior because it is too unhealthy for you to be around, you must set a healthy boundary with the person. Create some space. But what Accepting Communication does is empower you to speak with dignity and respect while setting that healthy boundary. It might sound something like this:

I love you, but when you _____ (fill in the blank with the un-acceptable behavior), I feel _____ (fill in the blank with your emotion). I don't feel strong enough to be around you. I'm willing to support you in getting help, but I won't support this behavior. We both deserve better.

Learning to be accepting of others means accepting yourself and your own mistakes, too—as big or as unforgivable as you may believe they are. You deserve peace of mind, no matter what you did or didn't do.

This is when we first begin to see true forgiveness show up.

When I use the term *forgiveness*, I'm referring to a conscious choice—mindfulness—to take back your power by letting go of your expectations of who you want the other person to be. Forgiveness is wisdom that impresses upon us that maybe "this" is how it needed to be in order for us to learn, grow, and expand our consciousness.

In this emotional space, we've come to terms with "what is." Forgiveness, therefore, isn't about change (although change often comes). Forgiveness encourages us to accept the person without accepting his or her behavior.

Forgiveness in application may sound something similar to this:

> I don't like what happened, but I know I can't change it. As difficult and challenging as this has been for me, I've been angry long enough. The gift of this experience is what I've learned about my Self and my ability to love. I forgive you.

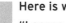 **Here is what forgiveness does *not* mean:**
"I agree with what you did" or "I invite you to do it again."

## FACING OUR SELVES

It reminds me of the overwhelming shame, guilt, and fear I experienced after not taking my fourteen-year-old daughter straight to the hospital one night when she came into my room complaining of stomach pain. It didn't matter that she was a high-maintenance child, that she often cried wolf, that it was flu season, or that she was getting her period the next day; I didn't listen to what she was saying, and as a result I almost wasn't able to be her advocate in time.

It was three a.m. when she climbed into bed with me. I asked her how bad her tummy hurt on a scale of one to ten, and if she could wait until the morning to go to the doctor. She said, "Ten, but yes, let's wait until the morning."

Who knew with this kid what a "ten" really meant? She'd said it so many times before . . . so I gave her Gravol and Tylenol and waited a few hours.

My husband went downstairs to sleep on the couch, and my daughter and I curled back up in bed and fell back asleep together. The next morning she got her period and vomited a few times, so I was sure that's all it was: menstrual cramps and the flu. I kept her medicated and sleeping for two more days. She didn't complain much again.

The third morning I knew something wasn't right. She got up to go to the bathroom, and she looked as if she'd lost ten pounds.

It was time to go to the hospital. She fought me the whole time: "Nothing is wrong!" she told me. "They won't even find anything. They'll just send us home!"

After taking her to our small country emergency room, the doctor said her white blood cell count was skyrocketing and decided to put her in an ambulance and send her to a larger hospital about thirty minutes away. After being stabilized at that hospital because she'd had an anaphylactic seizure as a result of an allergy (one we knew nothing about until then) to the contrast dye used in the MRI, the surgeon finally opened her abdomen up about twelve hours later and discovered her appendix had *already* ruptured.

After the operation, no one seemed overly concerned with her condition, but I could tell she was rapidly declining. By the next afternoon, I could see that she was struggling to breathe properly and was acting and saying bizarre things that didn't make sense to me. My fierce protective Momma Bear instincts were finally, *thank God*, kicking in.

No matter what the doctor said, I knew that something wasn't right—so I demanded a second opinion.

Apparently, my worries were on target.

The "second opinion" got straight on the phone with the Hospital for Sick Children (SickKids).

In an absolutely shocking whirlwind, a helicopter was immediately sent to transport my child to a team of waiting doctors in their ICU.

By one a.m., with my daughter slipping away, a surgeon told me to prepare myself for the worst. "She may not make it through the night," he told her father and me.

When we were finally allowed back in to see her a few hours later, she was on life support. Her lungs had collapsed, and her organs were shutting down. Her heart was racing out of control, and her fever could barely be managed.

Another operation was scheduled, and six drainage tubes were inserted into her body. Bags of ice were poured all around her, and constriction stockings were placed on her legs to try to stop the severe swelling. She was so swollen, you could barely recognize her.

SickKids is a teaching hospital; a large group of medical students travel from bed to bed and discuss each patient's individual situation. This meant that we were constantly listening to the doctors who stood around the foot of her bed reviewing the seriousness of her prognosis. Regardless of the fact that she couldn't speak (the ventilator tube was placed in her mouth and down her throat), she was old enough to understand how serious their concerns were. She was becoming increasingly despondent. Passivity was kicking in. She was beginning to lose her willingness to fight. I could feel it. She had stopped being aggressive—scribbling angry notes to me about different doctors and nurses. And this concerned me.

It was at this point that I realized I was her only advocate! She needed me to speak on her behalf. If something didn't feel right, I asked questions. At one point when they were debating a third surgery, I stepped in and disagreed. I asked them to give her a little more time for her body to do its own healing. The head surgeon agreed with me, saying, "Most mothers have an inner knowingness that more doctors need to respect." It proved to be the right decision.

Instead of letting her feel terrified and afraid of dying, I took the head doctor aside and asked him to stop talking about her as if she wasn't able to hear. Instead, I went back into the room and told her that things were turning around and looking up! She smiled and, for the first time since entering the hospital, gave me a thumbs-up.

I sat beside her day and night, reminding her of how strong she was and how well her body was responding. I insisted each day that she was improving, whether the numbers on the screens behind her bed indicated improvement or not.

After nearly a month on life support, my fierce, little fourteen-year-old left SickKids in a wheelchair, weighing less than seventy-eight pounds. Her spirit to live was astounding. And my spirit to protect her bonded us in a way that could never be questioned again.

Not to mention, God bless those doctors and nurses! They not only saved her life, they tried to assure me it could have happened to anyone. But deep down, I couldn't accept this. *I was my kid's protector, and she nearly died on my watch.*

It took huge courage to admit this to myself.

The doctor felt that being a competitive gymnast both

cursed and saved her. Apparently, her pain tolerance was so high from all her intense training that she could sleep through an appendicitis attack, yet without all the muscle she'd packed onto her tiny body, she wouldn't have made it. Her body fed off the muscle to stay alive.

But I couldn't help but wonder, If I had put her on tons of antibiotics for little coughs and simple colds while she was growing up, would the high dosage of antibiotics have saved her life when she really needed it most, or would she have become immune to the drugs, as so many children are these days? I also wondered, If I hadn't medicated her for two days on Gravol and Tylenol, would a simple appendectomy have been all that was needed?

It took me close to four years to forgive myself:

How could *I* have been so mindless?
How could *I* have screwed up so badly?
How could my daughter *forgive me* so easily?

I truly had no idea I was carrying so much shame, guilt, and post-traumatic stress until the tears streamed out of me for days as I kept listening to her favorite song, "Ride" by Lana Del Rey, as I wrote the pages of *this* book.

No wonder I'd gained nearly thirty pounds the year after! No wonder I poured myself into my work. No wonder I drank too much wine at night. Feeling all this pain was almost more than I could bear!

You're not always going to get it right. I guess that's why they say hindsight is 20/20. If you could change it, you would. But you can't.

The great news is that facing your buried stuff allows you to accept, let go, and heal. It allows you to forgive yourself in spite of yourself. It allows you to get on with your life. It allows you to get happy. It allows you to expand rather than contract.

What I can do now is listen to Lana Del Rey with a smile on my face. The suffering is finally behind me . . .

What a learning lesson: to forgive . . . *myself.*

## The Final Stretch

The first time I felt *love*—overwhelming, unconditional, infinite, pure, limitless, omnipotent love—was after my first child, Madelaine, was born; and then, of course, the expansion of my heart was widened even deeper when my second child, Julia, came into this world.

Up until that point, I had experienced what I thought was love. I easily expressed this wonderful emotion to others (or again, at least, what I thought love was). I certainly felt overwhelming happiness for many things in my life. But it wasn't until I held my baby in my arms for the first time that I was filled with an emotion that I can describe only as divine, holy, pure love.

Once I knew what real love felt like, I was able to begin comparing the ways I treated others—including myself—to the way I treated my children. Was I understanding, compassionate, and open-minded with my family, friends, employees, and coworkers? Was I able to set healthy boundaries for their sake as much as mine (remember, love doesn't mean that you say yes to everything!)? Was I able to let my partner be his own person with his own needs, wants, and opinions?

I realized the only way I could resonate in love was to re-contextualize my past into lessons and gifts that emboldened me to regain my childlike wonder, curiosity, imagination, interest, excitement, awe, trust, joy, and belief in life and in myself rather than continuing to see my past as a source of pain and suffering.

*This became my quest.*

I spent time each day taking myself through my own guided meditations, which were similar to the "Healing the Feeling" guided meditation I provided in Chapter Three. I also worked diligently to release my triggers by walking myself through the ten-step process previously described. I learned how to journal, and I did a lot of it!

I would remind myself throughout the day of what Loving Communication looked and sounded like until nonjudgment became my new norm. It took effort. I didn't always get it right. I still don't. But I realized there is always a kind and compassionate way of saying or doing anything that needs to be said or done.

This doesn't always mean other people will necessarily be able to receive what you're saying with love, if they themselves aren't resonating here.

When you love someone, you know the necessity of telling the truth. The secret is being certain that what you're sharing *is* necessary, and not just a statement of your opinion or one made to ease your own guilt. Sometimes love simply lives and let's live. This takes wisdom.

I will assure you that if you have children, there is no more important job *for you* than to make sure your kids know how loved, worthy, and special they are.

Although being a good mother or father is *not* necessarily the most important job in the world, *if* you are a parent, being good at it is number one. Other priorities can be a close second, but choosing yourself over your children is no more empowered than choosing them over you. All relationships—even parenting your children—have to be a win-win. Yes, you need to be good, first and foremost, but not at the expense of your children. Consider the familiar airplane analogy: if air pressure in the cabin should drop and you are traveling with small children, put your own mask on first before assisting them.

Here's the catch: You need to parent as the Adult Archetype and not as the Parent Archetype (and certainly not as the Child Archetype). When you raise your kids in an atmosphere of assertive, accepting, loving, joyous, and peaceful communication, they will grow to become emotionally empowered adults. Open-minded. Loving. Trusting.

If you do have children and they object to your newfound empowerment, be patient but not guilt-ridden. No codependency or enabling. Kids most often just need time to make sure we (them and us) are still safe . . . and that life is still safe. Reassurance works wonders, no matter what the age!

If you have younger children, you need to be especially thoughtful of their needs. You are their primary caregiver, and they are counting on *you* to get this right. Yes—you still have the right to your own life, and dreams but you gave birth to little beings who are counting on you to love, protect, and guide them.

If you have hurt your kids—whatever their age, even unintentionally, or if you have done things you regret or have a relationship with them that is at odds, you must make amends before you can resonate as the Adult Archetype. This is the law of the universe. It's the natural way of things. It is how we teach love. It is how we expand consciousness. It is the trickle-down effect. Part of healing your own wounds is letting your children know how much you love them—regardless of what you may believe they have done wrong. It's finding forgiveness.

Making amends doesn't mean one or two "I'm sorry(s). Let's move on." Sometimes serious cleanup is required, but it's worth it.

If more parents would get it right, the world would not be in the mess that it's in. I think the most important message we can show our children is this:

> Being "you" is the ultimate gift you can give the world!
> You, *alone*, are enough!
> Be your Self.

This is how love speaks. Love expands acceptance. Love seeks peace.

I also began to pay attention to the way I treated myself. I would wake up in the morning and ask myself, "What would a day of total acceptance and radical self-love look like?" The answers, when I really allowed myself to imagine them, were simple and effortless. Love inspired me to take care of myself, not just for my life—my joy and pleasure—but also for how I was showing up in the world and how I was treating others.

In this energy, we treat all living things, including animals and nature, with care, kindness, and respect. Some call it love fever. Others say that love is blind. These things I'm not entirely sure of; what I do know for certain is that love heals all things. Love heals us.

Love is about letting down our walls and becoming fearless. It is here that we experience life in an easy, effortless, content, faithful, forgiving, allowing, receiving, jovial, empathetic, thoughtful, kind way. We overflow with happiness because we are in the flow! We're in love with life, and life loves us back! We feel Creative Energy flowing through us. It invites and encourages vulnerability, honesty, and trust. It encourages goodwill, with the belief that everyone can leave the exchange feeling enriched.

Love is not the crazy, sickening, or obsessive feeling many people describe. This beautiful verse from 1 Corinthians best explains what love is:

> Love is patient, love is kind. It does not envy, it does not boast, it is not proud. It does not dishonor others, it is not self-seeking, it is not easily angered, it keeps no record of wrongs. Love does not delight in evil but rejoices with the truth. It always protects, always trusts, always hopes, always perseveres.

When you communicate with love, you let go of your personal desire, preconceived expectations, and preexisting agenda. There is no need or desire to control anyone or anything. By holding no one prisoner to guilt or to your expectations of them, *you feel free*. This is forgiveness fully expressed: acceptanace expanded.

When you are resonating at this level, you feel worthy, authentic, important, caring, giving, and whole—you are conscious. Mindful. Fully awake. Fully empowered.

No longer concerned about being right or proving a point, love is a wise, limitless, and unconditional guide for finding resolution and uplifting. Desire may be the root of all empowerment, but it certainly isn't the blossoming, fragrant flower opening for the first time! Love is the miracle of the butterfly leaving the cocoon. Love is freedom! Liberty! Magic!

This shifts us higher into Joyous Communication and then into the "cream of the crop" in terms of empowerment: Peaceful Communication.

Imagine for a moment that within your being, at any given time, you feel nothing other than pure gratitude and excitement about being alive. Present. Mindful. Festive. Blissful. This is what one feels at the level of Joyous Communication.

Most of us have joyous moments, but maintaining this level of emotional empowerment can feel like it requires an enormous expansion of consciousness. It doesn't, but perhaps this is why people and experiences that bring us joy, fun, and pleasure are so valued in our world—whether they be by way of entertainment, sports, arts, music, great food, literature, or something else.

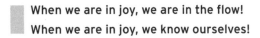

**When we are in joy, we are in the flow!**
**When we are in joy, we know ourselves!**

This is why laughter is the best medicine. Being in joy gives us so much *energy* that we no longer feel as though we have to force, demand, or manipulate anything or anyone ever again, in order to get our way. Things just work out for us! The bigger or more expansive our energy, the more powerful we feel! Joy, laughter, and love are the way.

In Loving Communication, we are happy. Not necessarily always getting our way, not necessarily always told we are right, but simply, truly, deeply happy.

Joyous Communication is a continual celebration of life . . . a celebration of the human spirit! When we are inspired, we are in spirit! We know our Real Self. We *are* our Real Self!

Joy is where all the Creative Energy or juices begin to flow from—where ideas come effortlessly; we have enough stamina to accomplish them, and problems resolve themselves. We simply have to show up and stay mindful of the signs! We listen to our gut instinct. We don't let the current take us, but we trust and move with it! Life becomes fun!

Joy intuitively knows that all will work out perfectly, as it should, as long as we stay in an expansive, trusting, mindful place.

*So what brings you joy? What lights you up? What makes your heart sing?*

The answers will give you peace. You can feel your truth within. It feels light.

Peaceful Communication can be very hard to recognize because it moves with the speed of the universe . . . with the speed of light. To the naked eye and to our sensibilities, the universe seems to move slowly, but Peaceful Communication actually resonates so quickly—or vibrantly—it appears to be inactive. Almost as though time stands still.

Think about it: Haven't you ever been so consumed in a project that you're surprised to see when you look up at the clock that hours have passed, rather than minutes? This is peace of mind. You've found your purpose. Your life has meaning. You are "lit up." You know who you are.

It reminds me of the scene in the fabulous movie *The Matrix*. Do you remember this 1999 sci-fi, prophetic classic in which Keanu Reeves plays a character called Neo—"the one" who is going to save the world?

If you saw this film, you'll never forget the scene where Neo is standing in the face of fear; as the bullets are flying, he begins to defy reality by moving so quickly that, to the viewer, he appears to literally "hang" in midair—peacefully, fearlessly, effortlessly.

Just watch a sunset: as slow as it may appear for the sun to drop gently below the horizon, the earth is moving at 1,675 kilometers per hour or 465 meters per second. That's 1,040 miles per hour. This magnificent level of energy is where great works of art, music, and architecture are created. You've accessed the highest realms of consciousness.

The quest is to maintain this level of empowerment! It is here where great feats are accomplished. Where fear is so far behind you that it feels utterly obsolete. This is where unexplained experiences and synchronicities occur. This is the ultimate in empowerment. This is where the magic happens!

When we are communicating from this place, our purpose works through us. We don't have to work for it—although to others, they may think we are working hard; we are in Creative Energy, allowing it to flow through us. Solutions become apparent, signposts are everywhere, resistance does not register, and everything unfolds the way it should. Life unfolds with trust, ease, joy, excitement, and happiness.

Dr. David Hawkins, author of *Power vs. Force*, claims that only 1 in 10 million people are Peaceful Communicators. "At this level," he says, "every thing is connected to everything else by a Presence whose power is infinite, exquisitely gentle, yet rock-solid."

This Presence is what Gandhi called the "force" in the quote that opened this book: "There is a force in the Universe, which, if we permit it, will flow through us and produce miraculous results."

It is what spiritual people call God. Peace is the most powerful Presence.

Peace is home.

This is who you *really* are!

■

Of course, transcending to Peaceful Communication takes mindfulness, although I hope by now you're excited about the prospect and can see why this work is so very much worth undertaking.

The next chapter will give you the tools to, gently but

effectively, clean up your unfinished business and heal old wounds so that you may become the greatest expression of who you are, and come home, to yourself.

It is time to become an empowered, happy, healthy, loving, peaceful adult!

# CHAPTER FIVE

# Who Am I?

**"BECOME"**

> We aren't meant to be perfect.
> We're meant to be whole.
>
> JANE FONDA

## Transcending Your Duality

For the majority of this book we have focused on our Dominant Emotional Archetype—the one we embody most to navigate through life; the one we think provides us with the greatest level of protection. But in order to have a dominant, we must also have a submissive. There is duality in everything.

Our Submissive Emotional Sub-Archetype(s) is the *most*

shameful or embarrassing of all the archetypes (in our mind)—the persona(s) we would do absolutely anything to avoid being or becoming. We do this by hiding, burying, or disowning this archetype in our subconscious mind.

The trouble is that by disowning these aspects of our humanity we develop inner conflict and self-loathing. We become anti-us. Anti-addict. Anti-martyr. Anti-ruler. Anti–chubby girl. Anti-troublemaker. Etc.

Mother Teresa was quoted as saying, "I will never attend an *anti*-war rally. If you have a peace rally, invite me." Achieving peace of mind, I imagine, requires a similar approach as achieving world peace. It will be realized only once we remove the "anti" aspect toward ourselves and replace it with acceptance, willingness, and understanding.

Our Submissive Emotional Sub-Archetype(s) is most often the opposite persona of our Dominant Emotional Sub-Archetype(s). It is this opposition that creates the conflict within. This is our most basic understanding of duality: the battle of our inner demons . . . or archetypes!

The underlying emotion behind all of this is fear. We fear our demons. We fear our shame. We fear ourselves. We fear what people think about us. We haven't been taught how to love ourselves—the good, the bad, and the ugly. Our self-love is conditional upon our being "good enough." We don't have peace of mind. We are forcing, gripping, pushing. Fighting ourselves as though we could ever win? We feel disempowered when we contract into our duality.

Just think about how much energy you exert—most likely unconsciously—trying to prove who you aren't, overcompensating for your supposed weaknesses and flaws, keeping yourself small because you are too embarrassed or afraid to face yourself.

Worried about the ways you've acted in the past, or the ways you've been taught never to be, the energy it takes to convince the world of *who you want them to see you as* eventually robs you of your power. It's inauthentic and exhausting. Managing yourself and all that fear becomes a full-time job. Not to mention, as we've previously discussed, "what you fear, you draw near."

In your own denial, you inevitably begin to attract and project your own unfinished business and buried fears into all of your relationships; unaware that everything that shows up in our lives is a mirror reflection of us. *Yes*—our relationships do nothing more than reveal *us* to ourselves!

Suffering arrives because it's time for us to look within to see where our own fear is drawing this experience into our lives so that we may see it, honor it, and heal it. Our abundance, sexuality, relationships, friendships, career, energy, health, income, vitality, joy—or lack thereof—is the *real* barometer of how in alignment we are with our Self—regardless of what our mind wants us to believe.

If any of these areas of your life are in disarray, rather than pointing the finger outward, why not look within to see where you have opposing inner views or beliefs that are creating conflict for you?

*Take a moment to consider what I'm saying:*

If you were honest with yourself, aren't there specific archetypes you actually view as more empowered, maybe even tough, sexy, or cool? Or others that are more loving, gentle, or caring? Are there some archetypes that, if someone referred to you as "one of them," you would be devastated and humiliated? The ultimate shame?

Tell the truth: Aren't there archetypes that you refuse to

believe you could ever be? Ones that you would do almost anything to prove you are not?

*Of course, there are! This is how shame works!*

> **Shame wraps around our ankles, whispering into our ears, that on some level we are no good.**

If you remember, in Chapter Three I explained how each of us grew up believing certain personality traits were unacceptable, unlovable, undesirable, and unwanted. Most likely, we (or someone close to us—a parent or sibling) were shamed for behaving in this way, so in order to avoid letting the world see us with these same qualities we made the decision to disown certain aspects of ourselves!

Our Submissive Emotional Sub-Archetype(s) can feel like an albatross around our neck—weighing us down, slowly destroying us. They are our deepest shame—our worst triggers. It is where our feelings of powerlessness, helplessness, and self-oppression arise.

A simple metaphor to explain this is to imagine you have many children: some are happy and easygoing, while others are more challenging. You even have one or two who are downright bad! So angered and embarrassed by the kids who behave in ways that are unacceptable, you lock those children in the basement, while allowing your lovely, happy-go-lucky kids to go outside, have fun, and play. In other words, some of your children are accepted and loved, while others are imprisoned and despised.

*Could you imagine doing that?*

No! You would never intentionally treat one child well and the other like a prisoner. You would love all of your kids, even when they're naughty! You may not like how they behave, but you love them! In fact, your most wounded children probably need your love and attention most!

And yet, this is precisely what we do to ourselves. We disown aspects of our humanity. We stop listening to or even caring for these personas. We deny some of our most basic needs.

Tired of being oppressed, our most disowned or Submissive Emotional Sub-Archetype(s) then occasionally bust their way out of the dungeon and, in rare episodes, confuse and shock the people in our lives—including our Self! We don't know who we are sometimes or why we act certain ways, just like Dr. Jekyll and Mr. Hyde! We've become the victimizer and the victim, the prosecutor and the prosecuted, the captor and the captive.

You have to learn to forgive, listen to, and love even the most shameful parts of you—for being human. You must heal the split.

You then have to forgive yourself for shaming yourself, if you are ever to learn to find love, peace, and forgiveness for yourself and others.

*This is why "your healing" must happen first!*

The question I pose is this: *What if the true way to transcend suffering is to accept it?*

Would you be willing to dig deep and figure out what you are most afraid of? Most ashamed of?

Would you be willing to accept yourself and love yourself—even in spite of yourself?

In the Introduction I shared that "when you take away choice, you take away empowerment." Choice is necessary for wholeness, which is why, I believe, duality is the spectrum of life!

It is our duality—the Child versus the Parent within us—

that allows us *the choice* to transcend into the Adult. Once we learn how to accept and then transcend this duality, we are able to know and "heal thyself"—fully and completely.

## Heal Thyself = Healthy Self

The fact remains: We are all things. We are the darkest night and the brightest sunrise. We are the enemy we fear and the friend we trust. It is our duality that creates the contrast that allows us to transcend into wholeness.

It is the willingness to choose to grow up and become the fully embodied Self; to own all of who we are—the good, the bad, and the ugly; to blow the lid off of exploitation, oppression, and fear; and to know that to be empowered we must embrace our darkest hours as deeply as we do our brightest moments.

It all matters. It all makes us who we are. There is no shame in being human. There is no shame in being flawed and imperfect. There is no shame in telling the truth.

It takes courage to do what must be done . . .

It takes courage to be an Adult in this world . . .

It takes courage to be your Self . . . *all of you!*

*This is the Emotional Edge!*

As one of my clients wrote to the group of people taking a 12-Week Telecourse with me based on *The Emotional Edge*: "Imagine what we will accomplish when this energy is free to create the lives we dream of!"

By embracing the Parent and the Child within us—one no more nor less important nor worthy than the other, and yet both equally needed and required—learning whatever lessons they are here to teach us, we become the fully integrated Self: authentic and whole.

As Debbie Ford shared in *Why Good People Do Bad Things*:

> Healing the split requires us to be firmly rooted in the reality that duality is central to our very nature. We couldn't know light unless we knew darkness; we wouldn't know courage unless we experienced fear. We would never recognize a kind heart had we not encountered a mean one. We could never know hope if we hadn't experienced the devastation of hopelessness. In this world of duality, the way we understand and gain wisdom is through comparison and contrast. So ultimately this journey is one of coming into balance with these seemingly opposing expressions of our humanity and learning to recognize the early warning signs that alert us when our inner world is out of balance.

Does "healing the split" mean I'm suggesting you should behave in disempowered and inappropriate ways and then tell yourself that it's okay or even acceptable?

*No*—I'm reminding you that when you allow yourself to fall into fear, shame, and guilt, you begin to contract into your duality instead of expanding into the wholeness of your being.

Shaming yourself for what you've been taught to believe is a "bad or unacceptable" version of you will only keep you disempowered. Fragmented. Broken.

We need to accept, forgive, and love ourselves rather than hate, despise, and humiliate. We need to learn from the most wounded parts of us. We need to expand our Emotional Sub-Archetypes by shining light on them, listening to what they need more or less of and then, encouraging them to ascend and expand rather than shrivel and die. *(Remember: Your Emotional Sub-Archetype(s) are a part of you. When you shame or disempower them, "you" too contract!)*

Expanding your Emotional Edges takes self-awareness,

courage, and willingness. We have to pull our heads out of the sand and wake up!

## My Personal Healing

You may remember that in the Introduction I explained that "although this book is nongender and many men and couples will benefit from reading it, I personally wrote this book for every woman who is tired of thinking about her flaws, fears, failures, and *fat*—those disempowered repetitive thoughts that are preventing you from becoming your greatest Self."

I am about to tell you why, while sharing one of my deepest fears:

I, like most women in our society, was taught that fat is the enemy, something to be especially ashamed of, and so at some point in my early life, I unconsciously made the decision to disown the Chubby Bubby. At the time, I didn't even know I was doing it.

Not unlike most girls, the women in my family constantly talked about their weight and how much suffering their body fat seemed to cause all of them. Appearance was a big deal in my family! We were the "anti-fat" and "pro-beauty" family! Being unattractive—particularly fat—was the great fear in our collective consciousness!

My grandfather made such a big deal about beauty that much of the time, probably without realizing, he pitted his six daughters against one another. "This" he'd say about my mother, when introducing her in front of his five other girls, "is my most beautiful daughter."

He would often do the same with me in front of all my cousins at various events and get-togethers. It created competition and envy. My long, blond hair hung past my butt, and he'd tell me to never cut it. My hair was my "crowning glory," he said; and being thin and beautiful was the ultimate prize!

The sad part is that even though every woman in my family was beautiful, I'm not sure if any of them could see what the mirror reflected.

What I do know is that if someone was to call any of us "fat" (even our own husbands), it was, quite possibly, the most upsetting and shameful thing that could be said—the worst of all the Emotional Sub-Archetypes! So much so that by the age of twenty-six, I found myself sitting in my rocking chair, sobbing . . . *because I was chubby.*

Not ironically, most of the women in my family eventually became overweight, although my mother went a different route and became obsessed with being thin, sexy, and fit. She worked out and dieted fanatically. She'd compete in up to ten bodybuilding shows a year, posing, tanning, dancing, oiling up, and strutting her stuff on the stage in a bikini. Fat was the enemy! And sex sells! The message was loud and clear!

In theory, one might believe that by shaming the Chubby Bubby versus accepting her, I would smarten up and start acting like the Thin Woman! And yet, the very opposite is what happened to me! These disowned parts of us always find a way to be heard!

In my case, eventually the Chubby Bubby barged her way out of the basement and demanded I pay attention to her . . .

When I look back, how on earth did I go from being the featured model in the *Ms. Galaxy* magazine of May 1994 to weighing well over two hundred pounds in February 1995? Yes, I had gotten pregnant and I hadn't lost all the weight. I know part of it was that, but there was way more going on and I knew it!

The inner battle I was facing was overwhelming: I hated and was ashamed of being chubby, so how could I love myself and stop shaming myself?

I couldn't!

I was always at war with myself. If I was losing weight, I felt good. If I was gaining weight, I was self-loathing.

Sure—I could say that I loved myself . . . *when I was thin*. I couldn't say the same thing when I was fat. I was on an emotional roller coaster based upon my weight.

Marianne Williamson describes the manifestation of our "Not-So-Thin-Self" in *A Course in Weight Loss*:

> This aspect of you only appears as large because she feels you are not looking at her, and she is trying to tell you something. She will not go away until she is accepted for who she is. Once she does feel accepted back into your heart, she will automatically respond to your desire that she manifests differently.

I realized that I'd built my protection as a sort of emotional holding tank similar to the septic tank in my country home. I didn't want all my crap to ruin me, so I mastered this ingenious way of burying my unhealthy emotions in my holding tank. *Just tuck it away over there. Who has time to deal with all this? I'd simply been given more than I knew what to do with. Smart, right?*

My weight—muscles and fat—became my armor—keeping out all the bad emotions. I didn't have to feel my pain, but I couldn't feel all the good stuff properly, either. I was *too* protected. I had a huge wall around my heart (and my body).

If you've ever seen a real septic tank, you'll know there is a manhole on top so that eventually all the crap can get cleaned out; otherwise, it will start spilling back into the house.

I needed to make peace with the Chubby Bubby. I needed to stop viewing her with shame, guilt, sorrow, fear, dread, and anger. I needed to dialogue with her in my journal.

I needed to honor and listen to her. I needed to apologize. I needed to accept her. I needed to learn how to love her.

My journaling looked something like this:

> Dear Crystal,
>
> I want you to know it sucks being the Chubby Bubby. In fact, I hate that you call me that! I hate the way I feel about myself. I hate not being comfortable in my own skin. I hate never having anything to wear. I hate that I have no willpower to change this! I hate always worrying what people think of me. I hate disappointing you! I hate causing us so much embarrassment and suffering.
>
> But the truth is, I never wanted to be in charge and run the show. I hate being in the limelight. I've done my best to take care of things . . . although clearly I suck!
>
> Besides, where have you been????
>
> If you are so enlightened and empowered, why haven't you been taking care of things?? Why am I under all this pressure? Why is it always my fault?
>
> I'm sorry I'm fat! I'm sorry you're embarrassed of me! I wish I could be different.
>
> Signed,
>
> The Chubby Bubby

*"Where have you been?"* the Chubby Bubby asked me. *"Where have you been?"*

For the first time, I finally knew who I was, and I wrote back from this place of accountability, understanding, and love:

Oh my love,

I'm so sorry. I've let you down. I've shamed you. I've shunned you. I've hurt you. I never meant to abandon, embarrass, or blame you. Please forgive me.

I went through a tough time in my teenage years and in my uncertainty, I forced you to take over. And that wasn't right or fair. I didn't know how to protect myself so I unconsciously made you become my protector.

But believe me, I'm here now. And I apologize for not stepping up and taking care of things sooner. I can only imagine how stressful it has been for you, trying to run the show. You're just a girl, trying to be a woman, trying to take care of us—and the lives we've created.

But I've got this now.

I trust myself. I know how to manage my life. I know how to manage my stress. I know how to set boundaries with people who want to hurt or take from me. I know how to manage my emotions. Trust me. I won't let you down again.

Besides, I need to thank you for stepping in when you thought I couldn't take care of things . . . when you thought I was too wounded. Too scared. Too broken. Thank you for doing your very best to protect us in the way you knew how. I'm not afraid anymore. I've got this. I love you. I'm sorry. Please forgive me. Please trust me.

Love,

Crystal
aka The Real Me

The Chubby Bubby and the Real Me dialogued back and forth in my journal, and as crazy as this may all sound, it was utterly liberating.

*This is how we find peace from all our broken pieces!*

It was amazing what the Chubby Bubby revealed to me!

She offered me insight and lessons about life . . . and mostly about me!

She is much more than a woman who simply eats too much; she is misdirected fear and shame manifested in the bodies of women all over the world. She is the woman who is taught to play it smaller in a larger body. The Chubby Bubby was keeping me unimportant, distracted, and—ultimately—disempowered. Besides, focusing on my fat (and my never-ending weight-loss struggles) gave me a full-time job! Who had time to live my purpose and passion? Who had time to shine brightly? Who had time to be the Real Me? Who had the time to write books, build an international coaching school, fall in love, get married, raise my children, *and be happy*?

Truth be told, the body shaming that happens to women who fall within the Chubby Bubby Sub-Archetype has another insidious side: what a great way to keep the women of the world small, preoccupied, and disempowered. *Focus on your fat, ladies!*

By allowing myself to be consumed with shame and embarrassment about my body, I never saw all of the lessons and gifts that the Chubby Bubby brought to my life. She taught me things such as how weighing myself was abuse. *"Would you do that to your own daughters each morning?"* she'd ask me in my journal.

Just picture it: *"Good morning, children! Come to the bathroom. It's time to get weighed. We need to know if Mommy is going to love you today. We need to know if today is going to be a good day."*

I also discovered hidden commitments the Chubby Bubby had made to some of my most favorite people, including one of my aunties, who showed me love when I was a child, my maternal grandmother whom I adored, and, of course, my role model, Oprah. They were all so kind, so loving, so beautiful, *and a little chubby.* In the mind of the Chubby Bubby, being fat had to make sense on some level—or why wouldn't these spectacular women be thinner? Being chubby worked!

I realized my Chubby Bubby also held a belief about fit, sexy women: they were conceited, neurotic, and troubled. Selfish! Narcissistic! Thoughtless!

Obviously, these beliefs are not true! But they unconsciously stemmed from how I'd been raised and what I experienced.

What a dichotomy I faced: being chubby brought shame but being thin brought fear. Both brought disempowerment, but which was worse?

The best part was when I realized there was no point in fighting with my Chubby Bubby any longer. I couldn't win! What we defend against, we create! She was the part of me that *I'd created* for my own protection! It was time to understand her needs (which ultimately, were my unmet needs) so that I could create a "win-win" relationship within. So I could be at peace.

In amazement, I discovered that as much as I thought the Chubby Bubby was my enemy, she came along precisely when I thought I needed her most: she was my protection. In my mind, it was for me to be a good mother, so the Chubby Bubby personality arrived alongside the birth of my first baby in February 1995. She offered me refuge from being the Charmer, the Warrior, and the Narcissist! She was my way of being more likable and less threatening *to others*. As her, I would never make my daughters feel less than me—especially during their formative teenage years when self-esteem is being challenged (a time when I struggled most with my relationship with my own mother). The Chubby Bubby would try desperately to put my husband at ease by making me less attractive, less sexy, less apt to cheat, and less apt to betray them all. I was passively despising my Self publicly in the hopes others would like her more. By playing it small, I thought I would fit in better with the moms at school, with the women at the gym, even with my own family. We could all bond over our self-loathing and extra body fat!

Once I really understood the role that the Chubby Bubby played in my life, she became less of an enemy and more of a gift. She was the part of me that needed more loving and less shaming. She showed me that I needed a safe place to share how hurt, abused, and angry I felt at my parents, at my abusers, at my family, at society . . . and at myself! *And on top of it all, she impressed upon me that she deserved love, pleasure, and affection—regardless of her weight!*

I listened, learned, and soon really began to love her. She was a part of me. She belonged in my heart, not in my dungeon.

Once I made peace with the Chubby Bubby who lived inside of me, I could literally feel the Real Me inside of the container that holds me—inside of my body. I could feel where *I* ended and my protection began. I not only felt her, I could hear her. She's where my Woman Energy resides.

The Real Me is happy, joyous, peaceful, accepting, and forgiving. She isn't angry, mistrusting, or afraid. She isn't insecure, comparative, or competitive. She's loving and lovable. Trusting. Courageous. Secure. Collaborative. Kind. Content in the skin she's in.

Now don't get me wrong, the Real Me is not a waif. She's not small-boned or petite. But she's not a bodybuilder or a fat girl, either. The Real Me is sexy, athletic, and strong. She is a goddess—regardless of my age!

Here, I'd spent most of my life sugarcoating my anger, avoiding my weaknesses and temptations, shaming my bad behavior (in myself and in others), and now, I was learning to listen to, accept, and even love all these wounded aspects of me.

I finally knew what the "connection" was that Bob Greene was always talking about: it's reconnecting with all our fragmented parts in order to surrender our suffering; carrying excessive weight is merely a manifestation of unhealed wounds—stored emotions that haven't yet found a safe place to be released. It has nothing to do with willpower, intelligence, or kindness. Our excess weight is housing our buried emotional suffering. I've learned the lesson. And I feel grateful for the gifts. I understand the disempowered, repetitive thoughts now—the misdirected fear that distracts and numbs us from the real stuff. And the best part is that I know that even the "real stuff" isn't real. It's all just distractions, disconnecting us from our Real Selves.

At some point, we have no choice: we have to process "our stuff" in a healthy way and let it go. We have to talk about *it*. If we don't, eventually *it* will stop us in our tracks: we will become ill, broken, angry.

Remember, the body is designed to *receive and release*.

It was time I did this with all *my* Emotional Sub-Archetypes—Dominant *and* Submissive. I needed to heal all the triggers that held an emotional charge for me.

My next stop was with the Addict, the Troublemaker, the Charmer, and, the worst of the worst in my mind, the Narcissist. I had to accept, and learn from, all these supposed shameful, self-centered aspects of myself in order to find balance, freedom, and happiness—to become the Light Worker that I am. (We will talk about the Light Worker in Chapter Eight.)

I understand if you feel like you aren't ready to dig up the emotional dirt and sift through it. I know it's scary to feel your feelings, honor your pain, and transcend your suffering but if you will let yourself, you can find your gold again, too!

Every painful experience has wisdom to be extracted. This is where the real healing takes place. Until this happens, you are always going to feel overloaded, overextended, overwhelmed, and/or overweight. You will always need to find a way to protect yourself from yourself.

I promise you: once you've gently dug up the misdirected fear and rerouted it, you'll have so much space left over for happiness and joy to infiltrate.

## The Real You

When I first begin coaching people, most times they have no idea that there are versions of them that "take over" in a sense, similar to what happens with someone who has "multiple personalities."

Now, of course, I'm not suggesting that any of us have a mental disorder, but we all put on different "masks" or "personas" in order to navigate different relationships. For example, you may be the Charmer with men but the Martyr with your children. *What matters now is that you realize none of these Emotional Sub-Archetypes define who you truly are. They are simply roles you've learned to play.*

Wouldn't it be wonderful to get to know the Real You—the person you were born to be? And to be the Real You everywhere you go, with everyone you're with?

Do you know how unique and important you are? Do you even know who you *really* are? Or have you forgotten where you buried your gold—your Real Self?

For many people, when I ask, *"Who are you?"* at my different retreats and workshops, I am often faced with a roomful of blank stares, searching eyes, and sometimes even tears.

Initially, I hear responses such as "I am a mother, a daughter, a sister, a wife" or "I am a writer or an actor." I've even heard "I am an old woman who has lived her life for everyone else. I am tired."

Once I tell my participants that I don't want to know who they are in relation to their family, occupation, income, gender, sexual preference, marital status, age, religion, culture, or zip code, I am usually greeted with more silence.

The answer to *"Who are you?"* may not be easy for you, either, because, perhaps, you've never been taught to differentiate your beliefs and the roles you play from the truth of who you are. In other words, you've learned to believe things about yourself that aren't true.

If you remember the story in Chapter One of the solid-gold statue covered in clay, you'll embrace the idea that no matter what you've been taught to believe about yourself, *you* can never lose your Self. You may bury him or her, but never lose him or her.

When you were a small child—before the world told you who you could be or should be—you had full access to your Self and to your unlimited potential, similar to the way a small pinecone contains all that is needed to grow into a magnificent pine tree. If given the right conditions to blossom, it will. Period.

You, too, contain all that you need in order to become a fully evolved, healthy, happy Adult. Your potential was planted inside of you before you were born. The difference between you and the pinecone is that you carry the soil, weather, and sun within you. Now, as an adult, you choose how you'll create your conditions. You decide whether you will blossom, regardless of the world around you.

The trouble is, for most of us we continue to play the role we learned in childhood. We continue to re-create the same conditions we grew up in. We do what is most familiar. Familiar comes from the word *family*.

To become a fully empowered Adult, we must access our Real Self—not the persona, mask, or archetype we've been taught to play.

To do this, I urge you to first consider whom you could be if you had never been bullied, wounded, betrayed, abandoned, hurt, abused, or neglected.

Whom could you be if you'd been taught only that who you are is already enough, and that you don't need to be, become, fix, change, or achieve anything else in order to be considered valuable, worthy, wanted, or loved?

Whom would you be if you never had to layer yourself in clay—in protection—in order to stay safe?

Think about it: If you hadn't been berated, insulted, or treated poorly ever, in your entire life, how would you feel about yourself today?

On the other hand, if you had only been encouraged, inspired, supported, and praised, who do you think you'd be? How would you feel about yourself? What would you believe about yourself? About love? Life? Happiness?

This is not intended to cast blame on anyone.

Our parents can consider the same question: Who would they be if they had never been wounded? And their parents (our grandparents) could ask the same. Although we can't change the past or undo our experiences, we can recognize our family legacies—our own patterns and self-limiting beliefs—and change them. We can heal our futures.

One of the ways that I help my clients access their Real Self is by using guided meditation. If you need help with this, please visit **www.TheEmotionalEdge.com** and download my meditation titled "The Real You."

## "THE REAL YOU"—GUIDED MEDITATION

Let's get started:

Begin by sitting in a comfortable chair.

Back upright. Breathing deeply, right down to your belly button.

Close your eyes and give yourself a few moments to become mindful and relaxed.

Let your shoulders relax down from your ears. Let your breathing deepen.

Wonderful!

Next, I want you to picture in your mind a "mini you" standing on a platform, similar to an elevator. When you feel ready, I want you to see yourself lowering down out of your brain and into your breath.

What I encourage you to do next is to reminisce back to a time when you felt really happy. It may have been the birth of your child, your wedding day, a family holiday, Christmas morning, or something as simple as standing on the beach watching the sunset. You may have different memories come up. Choose one. There is no competition.

Once you've decided on a particular event, allow yourself to feel it as fully as possible: Where were you? How old were you? Who were you with? What were you doing? How did you feel? What emotions might describe you in this moment?

Some sample words might be *loving, peaceful, calm, happy, joyous, trusting, patient, inspired, free, lighthearted, beautiful, relaxed, alive, adventurous, strong, magnificent, feminine/masculine, enlightened, excited, purposeful, powerful, connected, fulfilled,* and so on.

Think of at least five ways to describe your Self in this memory. What words instantly come to mind? Don't overthink it.

Remember these words so that you can write them down when you've finished this guided meditation. Say them to yourself again, one more time.

Wonderful!

Next, let's allow these emotions to magnify, intensify, and spread throughout your body. Try to feel your own happiness!

Breathe this good feeling in.

Take a few deep breaths to anchor these words, or emotions, deeply into your body, into your core.

Now you're going to reconnect with the part of you that is fully awake, sensual, strong, and potent, regardless of whether you have young children, haven't felt vibrant lately, or are getting older.

Depending on whether you are a man or woman, I want you to think of a Greek or Roman god or goddess: Aphrodite or Venus are good examples for women; Hercules or perhaps Zeus for men! What aspects of the god or goddess do you most admire?

Again, don't overthink this: What characteristics immediately come to mind? What qualities make this archetype so enticing and empowering to you? Notice how these god-/goddesslike personas represent passion, excitement, pleasure, adventure, fertility, sensuality, sexuality, beauty, virility, and strength! What parts of them do you most identify with? Again, remember the words so you can write them down, as well. Say them to yourself one more time. Anchor them into your body. Feel them.

Think of the other equally important facet of your Self that allows you to stay in balance and congruent with your highest or Real Self: the Saint or the Angel Archetype, maybe the Hero or the Knight in Shining Armor?

What qualities about these most respected archetypes inspire you most: *integrity, divinity, peace, truth, kindness, honesty, esteem, compassion, empathy, devotion, love, faith, trust, selflessness, protection, courage, sacrifice,* or *commitment?* Again, take a moment to be mindful of these words so you can write them down.

Feel them. Anchor them into your body.

Imagine what a person would be like who embodied all these wonderful characteristics that you've resonated with! Imagine the energy they would exude. The power. The presence. Their Emotional Age! No matter their Chronological Age, how empowered would they be?

Feel this feeling. Anchor it into your body.

Take a few deep breaths. Inhale. Exhale.

When you feel ready, gently bring your awareness back to the room.

Open your eyes, pick up your journal, and jot down all the words that came to mind: the five happy emotions, the god-/goddesslike qualities, and then the angelic or saintly virtues.

Now . . . here is the exciting news:

The words you've chosen are those that best describe the Real You! They are who you *really* are!

When you navigate your life from this emotional place, you fully embody the Adult Archetype. You become the greatest expression of your Self.

Again, this takes mindfulness to remind yourself of who you really are and not the lies you've been told or believe. I encourage you to write these words out as a Personal Truth Statement and read it often—at least once in the morning and once in the evening. It works even better if you look into your own eyes; feeling the words as you say them, until they become completely anchored into your core. (Remember, your brain creates beliefs based on repetition. You are retraining your brain for success, confidence, and empowerment! Remind yourself of who you really are many times throughout the day.)

For example:

I am loving, connected, purposeful, excited, peaceful, feminine, strong, sensual, angelic, and divine.

Once you've created your Personal Truth Statement, ask yourself if you feel connected to it. *Do you believe it about yourself?*

If not, that's okay! It doesn't mean that your Personal Truth Statement isn't true! You've just buried these parts of you so deeply that you need to allow them to come up out of the basement! It just means it's time to "heal the split" or expand the consciousness between your Real Self and your disempowered Emotional Sub-Archetypes. It is time to create space for greatness to blossom! It's time to be your Self!

## Healing the Split

Once we can find and own all the Emotional Sub-Archetypes we've embodied along the way, we can become empowered adults—whole and complete. To do this, we must invite all of "ourselves" back home, in a sense, for a family reunion—just without all the conflict and drama!

You may discover a very young scared child inside of you, along with an old angry Ruler, and every Emotional Age in between. It's as though, over the course of our lives, we've had trajectory-changing emotional moments—traumas and tragedies that left an indelible mark —prompting a new Emotional Sub-Archetype to emerge in order to protect us. The trouble is, once we are "done" with each particular archetype, we shove it down into the basement and then feel fragmented.

If you feel ready to become a fully integrated woman or man—healed, healthy, and whole—get out your journal and begin by asking yourself which Emotional Sub-Archetypes you most *resist*. I call these our *Submissive* Emotional Sub-Archetype(s).

Remember in Chapter Three when I asked you to identify the most undesirable or unacceptable behaviors in others, and then to stand in front of a mirror, look into your own eyes, and say over and over, "I am _____" (fill in the blank with the undesirable behavior)? Believe it or not, the qualities you most despise in others are *your* Submissive Emotional Sub-Archetypes.

I asked you to repeat the "I am _____" statement out loud until something in you shifts from feeling shame, fear, and anger into neutrality, even acceptance. Compassion. Understanding. Self-love. Forgiveness.

Before you can truly integrate and heal your Emotional Sub-Archetypes—dominant and submissive—you must first own them. You can't change anything until you acknowledge it.

If you haven't done the "I am" exercise yet, I urge you to go back and complete this ten-step process.

Doing the "I am _____" exercise neutralizes your deepest fears.

This is what it means to integrate the fragmented aspects of ourselves back into the wholeness of who we are.

Your next step is to have your own conversation with your Emotional Sub-Archetypes in your journal, beginning with your Submissive Emotional Sub-Archetype(s).

Here's the thing to keep in mind: *denial* (*d*idn't *e*ven *n*otice *I a*m *l*ost) will do everything in its power to prevent you from owning the most "horrible" of the archetypes (in your mind). Denial causes us to believe our own stories so we struggle with allowing ourselves to connect with or accept the archetypes we most resist.

*We convince ourselves there is no way this ugly aspect of humanity is buried deep in our unconsciousness!*

If denial happens, you will end up getting in the way of your own healing.

> Doing this journaling exercise takes a great deal of courage and willingness, but where there is a will, there is a way.

A willing person is an expansive person. A willing person seeks the truth over everything else. A willing person wants to find the answers. A willing person allows and learns rather than oppresses and controls.

Isn't it time to heal yourself? To face your shame, guilt, blame, sadness, fear, anger, and lack of forgiveness?

Get out your journal and allow the Real You and the Wounded You to write back and forth to each other. Let the Wounded You—your Submissive Emotional Sub-Archetype(s)—speak first. Give them a voice to express themselves. Think back to those trajectory-changing traumas and tragedies you've faced. Who was running the show back then?

*Questions you can ask might include these:*

- When did I decide to disown you? How old was I? What was happening in my life?
- Where are you buried? (See if you can feel the heaviness inside your body.)
- Why am I so afraid of you, your personality, and your needs?
- How old are you?
- What emotions do you feel?
- What are you here to teach me about where I am neglecting or hurting myself?
- Where do I need to embody a little more of you in my life?
- What Emotional Sub-Archetypes are *you* most afraid of me becoming? Why? What fears do those Emotional Sub-Archetype(s) stir up in you?
- What do I need to do to help you relax and allow me (the Real Me) to take care of things?

You may find your Submissive Emotional Sub-Archetype(s) have a lot of anger and sorrow that must be released. Don't deny or avoid doing this. Don't send them back to the basement! Be sure to acknowledge all their "should have beens," "could have beens," and "ought to have beens."

Write back to them.

One of the most important things that all humans need is to be acknowledged. Once we validate our wounded selves by listening to what they are telling us that we need more of or less of, they lose their power and the need to be seen and heard. So tell them what they've needed to hear; in essence, what you needed to hear when you were younger, afraid, scared, angry, or alone. Open yourself up to seeing your own blind spot— where you've forgotten to take care of yourself.

Tell your Submissive Emotional Sub-Archetype(s) that you love and forgive them. Say it out loud many times throughout the day. Use your own name when addressing yourself, i.e., *"I love you, Crystal. I forgive you for any mistakes you've made."* Wrap your arms around your body and give yourself a hug while you say it!

Even if this feels futile or silly at first, I promise the long-term effects will be profound. This is how you allow the wounded, constricted aspects of you to expand into acceptance, love, joy, and peace. This is how you'll find balance, authenticity, and freedom.

Be sure to notice your breathing as you do this. Whenever you feel yourself constricting and contracting into fear, you will immediately feel yourself holding your breath. Refocus on deep, expansive breaths. Doing so will instantly help shift you back up the Empowerment Spectrum.

Once you've made peace with the part of you that has been most buried—deeply suppressed—it is important that you find the opposite persona—your Dominant Emotional Sub-Archetype—and dialogue with him or her, as well. You'll probably feel more familiar with this persona. Your Dominant Emotional Sub-Archetype has been running the show—overcompensating for your Submissive Emotional Sub-Archetype. This archetype needs a voice, too!

This dominant part of you is tired; he or she has been in charge for far too long and for too much of the time. Give yourself permission to listen to and access this overly protective and most hurt place. It is time to chip away the clay and let the Real You expand—breathe! Shine! Smile!

Take your time doing this process. There is no rush. Continue to dialogue until you feel a sense of peace from within.

And when you start to feel yourself feeling disempowered again—frenetic, angry, or afraid—ask yourself these simple questions:

If I didn't have to worry what anyone thought of me (if it didn't make me a bad person, parent, child, friend, partner, lover, in-law, employee, boss, whatever), what am I feeling? What emotions are under the surface that I'm trying to suppress or avoid? What Emotional Sub-Archetype is trying to get out and be heard? What is this archetype worried about or afraid of? What do I need to assure him or her of?

And then, again, dialogue in your journal. Let your own inner wisdom speak to the wounded or fearful aspects of yourself. Acceptance is the key. Invite your fear out of the basement and give it a place to express itself. Fear loses its power when you shine light on it. This is empowerment.

And when you are done, thank your Emotional Sub-Archetype! No more shame or blame. This is what it means to "hold space" for your own healing. The only way to find wholeness is by accepting "yourself" the same way you would a wounded child.

*Yes*—give gratitude for their lessons! Give thanks for their unhappiness! They are aspects of you that will help keep you in balance if you'll listen to them rather than oppress them whenever things become painful or stressful. The secret is to recognize the early warning signs that show you that you feel out of balance before you begin to contract into your fear and duality.

Slowly but surely, you'll realize you are becoming healed and whole. Authentic. Empowered. You'll love yourself, even in spite of your flaws. You'll maybe even stop noticing them! You might even find radical self-love becomes easy and natural for you!

In the future, when you recognize your Submissive or Dominant Emotional Sub-Archetypes rearing their little "personas" again, causing chaos or suffering in your life, acknowledge them. Don't deny them. Dialogue with them:

> **What you resist, persists.**
> **What you reject, you project.**
> **What you accept loses power and diminishes.**

"Peace of mind" is the best way to describe this experience.

Finally, it is important to note: just as I mentioned with some of the other processes that I've encouraged you to do in earlier chapters, reading the above exercise and actually doing it are not the same thing. Until you dialogue with both your Submissive and Dominant Emotional Sub-Archetype(s) in your journal, you cannot imagine the freedom you will find.

Give your Self this beautiful gift!

## Using Your Body to Guide You

One of the things I've already mentioned is how human bodies have their own "truth barometer," almost like an internal compass or internal GPS (global positioning system) guiding us:

> **Red light:** *Stop!*
> **Yellow light:** *Proceed with caution!*
> **Green light:** *Go!*

Your body is so brilliant that I'm going to show you a simple exercise that you can do anywhere, anytime, to know the truth. Here's how it works:

On a blank piece of paper, write down ten things you know

for certain to be true. (You must write them down. And they must be facts rather than opinions.)

At the end of the ten statements, write down one question you want an answer to—but it must be written as another factual statement.

Then, one by one, say each statement out loud. For example, here is what I did when I had a question about my diet:

1. My birth name is Crystal Nicole Andrus.
2. My date of birth is December 11, 1970.
3. I am a Sagittarius.
4. I was born in Toronto, Canada.
5. My eldest daughter's name is Madelaine.
6. My youngest daughter's name is Julia.
7. I am married to Aaron James Morissette.
8. I write books.
9. I have blue eyes.
10. I am five feet six inches tall.
11. My body feels good after I eat wheat.

*Wait. Did that last statement feel like truth? Did it feel the same as the others?*

When I repeat: "My body feels good after I eat wheat," I feel something physiologically change in my body. The truthful statements all felt natural—my body was at ease—but when I spoke the last statement, I felt an instant, yet gentle disconnect within my body; a feeling—a gut-instinct—but not one that I need to become emotional about.

*Why don't you try this for your Self and see what your "truth barometer" tells you?*

Go ahead! Write down ten things you know for certain to ·

be true. Then write down one question that you want an answer to in the form of a factual statement.

Read your eleven statements out loud and feel the truth! Your body knows. *And once you know, you know.*

In time, you'll begin to know the answers to your own questions so quickly that you won't need to write ten factual statements first. Your body will know what the truth is for you because your body knows.

Your body knows if you've been overeating or undereating.

Your body knows if you've been indulging in too much alcohol or fast food.

Your body knows if meat, wheat, or dairy doesn't work with your system.

Your body knows if you haven't been moving enough.

Your body knows if you've been mindful or mindless!

The clearer, healthier, and more empowered you are, the easier it is for you to feel the truth!

When you don't do what you know, you'll feel out of alignment. Frustration sets in. And shaming yourself won't fix anything! In fact, shaming yourself will only shift you further out of alignment—creating passive, heavy, helpless emotions. Start listening to and loving your body and you will never need to diet again!

The problem for many of us is that we can't properly access our internal GPS because of all the distractions going on inside of us—excessive food, chemicals, preservatives, pesticides, painkillers, caffeine, sugar, nicotine, alcohol, drugs, or any number of the different things clogging and bogging down our insides; or a lack of vitamins, minerals, nutrients, and water.

Not to mention, every time we get pulled down into a fearful or anxiety-producing situation we create chemical reactions within the brain and body—almost instantaneously.

Remember, emotions create chemicals. The brain produces more than fifty active drugs—some far more powerful than morphine. The relationship between emotions and the body is now called mind/body medicine.

Here is the crucial part in this:

> Whatever chemicals our body has become accustomed to, it craves more of those same chemicals, no differently than the way a smoker craves another cigarette.

Chronic, fear-based chemicals damage our bodies, lowering our immune system, depleting our endocrine system, and slowly destroying our health. For example, if you've been under stress for an extended period of time, your body has become accustomed to the stress hormones racing around in your system. If your life starts to become less stressful, your body will go into withdrawal. Nothing but more stress will give the "hit" of adrenaline you need to maintain your emotional baseline.

This is partly why we continue to sabotage ourselves, even when we know better! We've disconnected from our internal GPS. Instead, we've become physically *addicted* to our emotions—even the disempowering ones!

One may ask: How is it possible that someone could become addicted to grief, as an example?

It's possible because the memory of the deceased loved one triggers not only the pain of loss but also a feeling of love and connection. In fact, science confirms that the brains of people experiencing long-term grief showed activity not only in the *pain* network of the brain but also in the *reward centers*. This pain/reward dichotomy is why we get stuck in a loop of disempowerment, addictions, and suffering. We are addicted to our biology!

*Do you get this?*

Every time something dramatic, painful, or dysfunctional happens, you get a *hit of drugs/chemicals/hormones* that temporarily makes you feel a sense of normalcy or familiarity. Relief. But within no time, you need that *hit* again.

Without realizing it, you've become drawn to and may even start creating drama and dysfunction. You stay stuck in unhealthy relationships without even trying to fix them. Escaping your problems feels next to impossible because you can never escape yourself. You feel powerless to your own biology.

**Do you see why this isn't about willpower?**
**You are not weak or stupid!**
**You're addicted!**

You can be a great person—a wonderful, loving, kind, compassionate, smart adult—whose body is addicted to suffering, stress, and fear. Your body is confused, unsure of what to do or how to get back onto the right path. It has become addicted to the chemicals your brain has been consistently releasing; as well as clogged by the unhealthy food, drinks, and air you consume.

*Becoming an Empowered Adult, therefore, requires a three-part process:*

1. Detoxing physically and emotionally from stress, drama, and dysfunction.
2. Healing and releasing old emotional wounds held within the body.
3. Nourishing your Self with healthy foods, healthy relationships, and healthy thoughts.

Think about this: the first four letters in the word *healthy* are *h-e-a-l*. In order to be healthy, we must "heal thyself." No coincidence, either, that the first three letters in the word *diet* are *d-i-e*.

If you struggle with your weight, I'm here to tell you: never diet again! Dieting is about repression, oppression, aggression, shame, guilt, blame, and self-loathing. It doesn't work. Never did. Never will.

Instead, you are going to learn to listen to your body, uncover your self-limiting beliefs, heal your buried stories, release the stagnant energy, and nurture yourself with authentically good food, good moods, and good company!

In my case, I can honestly say that I love my body now and my body loves me—no matter what my weight, wrinkles, or waistline has to report. Beauty is in the eye of the beholder. I love myself—all of me.

The important part to remember is that your body is designed to receive *and release*, both physically and emotionally. When you eat something, for example, your body absorbs all the nutrients and then flushes out the rest. It is not designed to hold on to unneeded materials or waste. *Your emotional body is the same.* You are designed to experience relationships, absorb the lessons, and *let go* of the rest.

The trouble again is how few of us were taught how to feel, process, and then let go emotionally. Our bodies instinctively process our food and expel what we don't need, but we have to actively work to process our emotions in the healthiest way possible. If we don't, we end up holding on to all of our memories, experiences, suffering, and stories.

The truth is, most of us bury our most painful experiences deep in our psyche—and over time, these suppressed experiences begin taking their toll on us emotionally, physically, mentally, and even spiritually; we then wonder why, over time, we start feeling bogged, clogged, and exhausted. In a sense, think of your body as your Secret Keeper—each buried tale holds a gift in among all the pain and suffering.

But we aren't sure what to do . . .

Our GPS seems to be broken.

We can't feel our "gut instinct" anymore.

We're clouded. Disempowered. Mistrustful.

We can't trust ourselves, either. Life feels overwhelming.

Troubles are monstrous. We're weighed down. Stuck in the muck.

This is what happens when we use up such an enormous amount of energy to hold on to our crap!

■

In the next chapter, I will outline specific ways you can help keep your body—your truth barometer—in its healthiest, most empowered state so that you can continue to feel, heal, and evolve.

# CHAPTER SIX

# Conduit of Consciousness

## "CONNECT"

> When an inner situation is not made conscious,
> it appears outside as fate.
>
> CARL JUNG

## Path to Feeling

One of the most important things I remember hearing Bob Greene say while listening to his *Make the Connection* audiobook way back in February 1997 (the night before I began writing in my *first-ever* journal) was that our body represents our life. He encouraged us to stand naked in front of a full-length mirror to see what our body was telling us: "You could be better. You could be worse," he said. "But your body, right now, represents your life."

*Talk about blowing the lid off denial!*

Some eighteen years later, I still trust Bob's philosophy; however, I've learned that instead of seeing ourselves as we *really* are, we see ourselves *through the lenses of our Dominant Emotional Archetype.*

As I mentioned earlier, the Parent Archetype feels that spending too much time at the mirror is superficial. If those who embody the Parent Archetype do eat well and exercise, it is simply for the purpose of living longer and staying healthy so they can take care of their loved ones. Most often numb, living only from the neck up, the Parent Archetype is disconnected from their physicality . . . and sexuality.

Those who embody the Child Archetype have a very different relationship with their body than the Parent Archetype. The Child Archetype is so emotional that they either rebel completely against their body or obsessively think about making aesthetic improvements. The even bigger trouble with the Child Archetype is that nothing is ever middle of the road for them: Binging or abstinence! Marathons or coach potato! This archetype is all about extremes!

Those who embody the Adult Archetype, on the other hand, are connected to their body in a deeply physical, spiritual, and sensual way. With a healthy self-image and desire to take care of themselves (and others), these individuals focus on listening to and trusting the messages their body gives them. They realize their body is not *who* they are but rather is the container that houses their spirit. Without a strong and healthy body, nothing else in their lives can work as well, either.

As discussed in the Chapter Five, your body is your truth barometer. If you are having trouble feeling your body's messages, I want you to begin by asking yourself some basic questions that can help you become more mindful:

Can you feel when you are hungry, or are you always munching? Do you feel when you are full, or do you tend to eat until it hurts? Can you sense when you are tired, and do you wake up when you've had enough sleep? Do you feel sexual urges and desires? Are you able to orgasm easily? Do you cry when you are sad? Do you laugh often throughout your day? Can you breathe easily and deeply?

Your body is your closest trustworthy instrument—*your best friend*: you'll want to start listening to it because it is your *most important tool* for staying vibrant, healthy, happy, strong, and empowered. One of the easiest ways to know what your body needs is to ask yourself this question each and every morning, "What would a day of Radical Self-Love look like?"

Your own inner wisdom knows exactly what you need: more sleep, less stress, more play, less junk food, more love, less suffering, etc.

The following tips are a guideline that *all* human bodies need in order to stay healthy and strong. These will help you to stay more "tuned in":

## Your Physical Needs

I'll never forget the perfect quote I read back in 1997 by Diana K. Roesch. It was in a beautiful little book called *Simple Abundance*, written by Sarah Ban Breathnach. This book traveled with me throughout the first year of my transformational journey.

> A woman's relationship with her body is the most important relationship she'll ever have. More important than husband, lover,

children, friends, colleagues. This isn't selfishness—it's just fact! The body is, quite literally, our vehicle for being—for giving, for loving, for moving, for feeling—and, if it doesn't work, it's fairly certain that nothing else in our lives will work, either.

I couldn't agree more. And in the years since I first read that beautiful observation, I have developed a simple but life-changing prescription for improving my relationship with my body that allows for me to be more expansive, energized, empowered.

I highly encourage you to incorporate this process into your life starting now. Be ready to be astonished at what happens! Here are my top seven steps for keeping your vehicle as high resonating as possible:

1. Drink a minimum of sixty-four ounces of pure, alkaline, high-mineral, nonchlorinated water daily.
2. Stop counting the calories in your food and start paying attention instead to the chemicals in what you eat!
3. Get your sweat on daily: move your body!
4. Get more sleep, please!
5. Have more fun!
6. Get outside more often—experience nature every day!
7. Create a Sacred Space.

## DRINK MORE WATER

Water is the carrier of all things in your body. It is one of the greatest energy conduits on earth. With lightening speed, energy is transported through water!

In my opinion, water, *not wheat*, is the staff of life. Your body is about 70 percent water. You were created in water.

At the time of your birth you were approximately 90 percent water. By old age, you'll be about 50 percent water.

Water loss equals aging, exhaustion, and a whole other slew of health concerns from aches and pains, migraines, bloating, water retention, foggy brain, obesity, etc. By the time you feel thirsty, you're already dehydrated.

The real trouble is what we are doing to our fresh water supply—*the world's drinking water.* Either so dirty or so depleted, we now have to add so many hazardous chemicals just to make it safe for consumption that we are hurting ourselves in a massive, long-lasting way. What kind of drinking water will our great-great-grandchildren have? What about the many food sources that are obtained from our oceans and lakes? Pregnant women are now advised to avoid eating many fishes that were once ideal protein sources!

Not only are we filling our bodies up with poisons, the chemicals needed to clean our contaminated waters are bleaching and depleting all the minerals from our drinking water—*minerals that keep us young, healthy, and vibrant.*

On top of it, the soil that our farmers grow our vegetables in, year after year, has also been depleted of minerals. Unless you are buying organic, you aren't getting the nutrients that your grandparents got. Period.

Did you know that without minerals our bodies cannot absorb or assimilate vitamins? Without enough minerals in our systems, we become acidic, an environment that is the breeding ground for almost all diseases.

Studies done by Linus Pauling, two-time Nobel Peace Prize winner, suggested that we can trace every sickness, disease, and ailment to a mineral deficiency in the body.

Drinking eight glasses daily of clean, healthy, mineralized, alkaline water is the number one most important thing you can do for your health, energy, and personal empowerment.

When you first start to drink more water, you will have to urinate more often, because your body will react like a dry sponge. Ever notice how a dry sponge can't absorb much liquid, but once it's wet, it can keep soaking up more and more?

Continue to drink clean, pure water until the urinating normalizes. You'll probably notice that your skin looks supple, fresh, and hydrated! The constant bathroom breaks will be short term. The long-term payoff, however, is exponential.

If you're a soda, coffee, even juice drinker, I'm going to give you a little bit more of a challenge. Every time you have a drink that is *not* water, be sure to "chase it" with a glass of water! Over time, you'll want to limit all caffeine drinks and reduce alcoholic beverages.

My most important request, however, is to stay away from all carbonated beverages, even soda water. Carbonated beverages are highly acidic and leach minerals, specifically calcium and magnesium, from your bones, DNA, and brain; plus, they're filled with chemicals you can't even pronounce! A body low in minerals becomes a breeding ground for disease.

Please visit **www.TheEmotionalEdge.com** if you want more information on ways to obtain clean, healthy, mineralized, alkaline water.

## EAT TO THRIVE

In the last hundred years we've had incredible advances in science, and although many of them have been brilliant in aiding mankind, there are equally disturbing consequences about the effects of some of these so-called advancements that include, but are not limited to, GMOs, pesticides, processing, preservatives, sweeteners, glucose-sucrose, high fructose corn syrup (which is in almost every packaged food, and 90 percent of all corn comes from GMOs), colorants, sulfites, poisons in our water and air, hormones in our meat and dairy, not to mention the excessive use of medicines, antibiotics, and vaccines. We're now facing the gamut of damage we've done to ourselves.

The Immune Disease Institute, a division of Harvard Medical School, reports:

> Worldwide there is a rising incidence of polygenic diseases, which include type 1 diabetes, multiple sclerosis, autism, asthma, and celiac disease (gluten sensitivity). Incidence of type 1, or juvenile, diabetes is increasing 3 to 5 percent per year, while celiac disease may now affect five to ten out of every thousand Americans.

You can't hurt a part of the whole and not hurt the whole. We've messed with Mother Nature, and now we're damaging ourselves. The extremely disturbing part is the number of our food-manufacturing companies that make massive profits by engineering food to be so "rewarding" to the brain that we are willing to damage ourselves for the sake of the "taste-bud payoff." This is known as the "food reward hypothesis of obesity." It means we want to keep eating, even though we're full. We crave more of the chemicals in the unhealthy foods that we've become addicted to.

Studies reveal that most processed foods are filled with chemicals that cause a *hyper-rewarding* experience for those who consume them, which effectively short-circuits the brain against overconsumption. Engineered foods are literally hijacking our minds and destroying our health. Just as we become addicted to our own emotional chemicals (adrenaline or dopamine, for example), we can become addicted to the chemicals in foods that aren't good for us, which clog the body's ability to feel and heal itself. Our brain becomes wired for eating more! The food is too addictive to stop ingesting!

So forget counting calories! Forget dieting! Just go back to the basics: if Mother Nature made it, eat it! Your body will know exactly what to do with food that came from the earth. You won't get fat. You won't get sick. And you won't get bored, if you learn how to cook it well!

Now, if this sounds blah to you (ugh, who wants one-ingredient foods, *right?*) commit to eating out once a week at a fabulous "health conscious" restaurant in your community. You'll be shocked that organic, free-range, vegetarian, or even vegan meals can make your mouth drool and satisfy your taste buds, all the while healing your body!

I guarantee that after enjoying a few downright delicious, healthy meals (that will leave you feeling energized afterward), your thoughts will change about healthy eating and you'll realize that, with a little effort, you, too, can easily make the most scrumptious meals at home with one-ingredient foods.

Yes—it takes more time to prepare a great meal, but what's the big hurry? You can make the experience of cooking a celebration of life.

Pay attention to how your body reacts after eating meat, wheat, dairy, sugar, sodium, MSG, nitrates, and all other processed foods. You may find eliminating these items, one at a time, over a two-week period will show you exactly what your body likes and doesn't like. Trust your body. It knows!

If you're struggling with your weight, I recommend that you stay away from starchy, heavy, "white" carbohydrates: bread, potatoes, pasta, and rice, and of course, sugar! The body thrives on lean protein, fiber, and colorful vegetables!

Stick with single-ingredient foods, those found around the outside edges of your grocery store, and you'll look and feel fabulous! Eat the freshest food possible! As soon as a fruit or vegetable has been picked, it begins losing nutritional value. This is one of the reasons I love having my own vegetable garden and fruit trees at my home. Bite into an organic tomato just picked off the vine and you'll know exactly what I'm talking about!

If you do buy a packaged food, look at the ingredient list. If it contains anything man-made, put it back. The ideal is to eat free-range, organic (non-GMO), one-ingredient foods.

## MOVE YOUR BODY

Plato wrote: "In order for man to succeed in life, God provided him with two means, education and physical activity. Not separately, one for the soul and the other for the body, but for the two together. With these two means, man can attain perfection."

As a kid who grew up playing competitive sports and doing track and field, I know that when I'm active, I'm happier! No questions asked!

Whether it's putting on my favorite music and dancing feverishly around my living room, speed-walking on the treadmill, getting outside for a jog, or connecting to my Self during a quiet yoga session, absolutely nothing in my life can surpass the energy I get from moving my body. And yet, here's the crazy part: *I still fight it!*

*Yep! Even I do!*

Who has time to run on a damn treadmill? Besides, where the hell are we going? Why should we practice dance steps or run around a court, hitting a ball or defending a net?

*Why?* Because it helps give us the Emotional Edge!

In fact, science is now showing us what we already know: exercise makes us feel better! But most of us have no idea why!

We assume it's because we're releasing endorphins, venting stress, or increasing energy, but the real reason we feel so good is because of what exercise does for our brains! It turns out that neuroscientists have discovered that "moving our muscles produces proteins that travel throughout the bloodstream and into the brain, where they play pivotal roles in the mechanisms of our highest thought processes!"

John J. Ratey, MD, wrote a national bestseller called *Spark*, which is undoubtedly one of the leading books on the revolutionary new science of exercise and the brain. "Exercise," Ratey says, "is like 'Miracle-Gro' for our brains":

> In today's technology-driven, plasma-screened-in world, it's easy to forget we were born movers—animals, in fact—because we've engineered movement right out of our lives. Ironically, the human capacity to dream and plan and create the very society that shields us from our biological imperative to move is rooted in the areas of the brain that govern movement. As we adapted to an ever-changing environment over the past half million years, our thinking brain evolved from the need to hone motor skills. We envision our hunter-gatherer ancestors as brutes who relied primarily on physical prowess, but to survive over the long haul they had to use their smarts to find and store food. The relationship between food, physical activity, and learning is hardwired into the brain's circuitry. But we no longer hunt and gather, and that's a problem!

We no longer hunt and gather. And this *is* the problem—in more ways than one!

Unfortunately, as we sit on our butts each day, working longer and longer behind computer screens, racing to the drive-thru to grab dinner, and then watching TV during the evening, we're losing our Evolutionary Edge. We've made our lives so easy that it's become incredibly complicated to nourish ourselves—our brains, bodies, and emotions—with what we need to "expand." Exercise, literally, makes us smarter, happier, and healthier!

Intense bursts of cardio exercise prove to be the most effective. Here we see huge improvement in those who struggle with ADHD (attention deficit hyperactive disorder), addictions, depression, learning difficulties, and aging, as well as for many other symptoms.

Personally, my entire life changed as I created a new habit of waking up each morning, tying on my running shoes, and hitting the pavement. The act of taking control of my body changed my entire life. Heading out, day after day, to exercise, no matter what the weather, is what woke me out of my unconscious mindlessness—my depression, my unhappiness, and my emotional eating.

It's simple physics: a body in motion stays in motion; a body at rest stays at rest.

Yet, how quickly we forget about that "feel-good" state that both exercise (and sex) bring to our body, mind, and spirit—hormones balancing, endorphins surging, metabolism revving, mental circuits supercharging, mood lifting, confidence growing, cravings for alcohol and junk food being reduced, and body fat diminishing!

We get used to our static lifestyle; we get used to getting by doing as little as possible. We avoid engaging our physical bodies even when we know that doing so will make us feel better.

But here's the big thing: you cannot embody the Adult Archetype and not move your body a minimum of three times a week—and five to six times is ideal. Exercise is the ultimate cleanser, flushing every cell in the body, removing stagnant energy—emotionally and physically. It gives us energy, vitality, and confidence. It improves our state of mind by creating an inner environment conducive to learning! Plus, it balances our hormones, prompting the release of feel-good endorphins! Exercise may as well be Mother Nature's Prozac!

There have been fewer people moving their bodies—which evolves our motor skills and brain—in the last hundred years than ever in the history of the world, and not coincidentally, we now have more illnesses, diseases, and obesity than ever before. Sure, we've improved infant mortality and increased life spans, but that doesn't mean we're healthier as a whole.

The great news is that finally the American Medical Association (AMA) is officially taking exercise seriously. In his inaugural address in 2007, Ronald M. Davis, the president of the AMA, encouraged his members to help each and every patient plan an exercise regimen!

(Note: It's hard to believe, but up until 2007, doctors— even psychiatrists—were never offered a course on physical activity or nutrition during their medical studies; pumping out prescriptions was their primary focus.)

Still, things must change! We must become the advocates of our own health. We must become physically empowered! Exercise is going to help keep us young, vibrant, and empowered! Some easy ways to incorporate exercise into your life is to think back to when you were a child—what activities were you most interested in doing simply because you had fun? Make a commitment today to start engaging in similar types of movement. If you loved dancing, put on music and dance around your home. If you loved sports, join your local YMCA and find a pick-up game of basketball or tennis. If you weren't very active as a child, make a commitment to get out walking every day.

## MORE SLEEP, PLEASE!

Why we sleep remains a scientific enigma! No one knows, yet, just why we need to sleep!

There are many theories—from our need to "restore" what is lost in the body while we are awake to compelling new research called "brain plasticity," whereby sleep (or a lack thereof) changes the structure and organization of the brain.

Although these theories remain unproven, what we do know is that if we go without sleep for too long, we become walking zombies! And walking zombies are not emotionally empowered!

As I stressed in my first book, *Simply . . . Woman!*:

Ask any mother with a newborn baby how jubilant she feels after many nights of little or no sleep. I remember when my children were babies, thinking, "I love my kids so much. Why do I feel unhappy?" Well, I was exhausted most of the time! I think a lack of sleep played a bigger part in my frustrations than postpartum depression did.

The average adult requires seven to eight hours of uninterrupted sleep every night—are you getting enough? A lack of sleep will increase your susceptibility to illness, and is frequently linked to car crashes and industrial accidents. It will make you irritable, exhausted, and even depressed. Sleep is also the time that our anti-aging hormone (HGH) is released. Without sleep, we're inhibiting our HGH, thus speeding up the aging process.

The following sleep practices can dramatically improve your snooze:

1. Get a comfortable mattress and pillow.
2. Stick to the same bedtime and wake-up time, seven days a week.

3. Avoid taking naps.

4. Get your sweat on. Exercise daily.

5. Keep the temperature in your room between 60 and 67 degrees. It's easier to sleep in cooler weather.

6. Turn off the lights—completely—or wear a sleep mask! Your closed eyes should be free of any light.

7. Avoid heavy meals in the evening.

8. Reduce or eliminate alcohol.

9. Consider taking a small dosage of natural melatonin thirty minutes before bedtime.

10. One final suggestion I'd love you to adopt before you go to sleep at night: Drink a glass of water, then lie flat on the ground or on your bed and place your legs above you, propping them against the wall or headboard. This is a wonderful exercise to help with circulation, increase blood flow back to your heart, and help eliminate toxins and reduce water retention. Drink a glass of water just before to help this releasing experience and to flush your system. What a wonderful night's sleep you'll have!

## HAVE SOME FUN!

Think about how good you feel after a relaxing vacation, a fun night out with girlfriends, or even an exciting new experience. Pretty great, right? You probably feel rejuvenated and refreshed, and you may even ask yourself why you don't do things like that more often. Well, I'm here to tell you that you should!

I recently had the pleasure of watching the Ted Talk by author and psychiatrist Stuart Brown, MD, called *Play Is More Than Just Fun*. As a pioneer in research on play, Dr. Stuart Brown says, "Humor, games, roughhousing, flirtation and fantasy are more than just fun. Plenty of play in childhood makes for happy, smart adults—and keeping it up can make us smarter at any age."

It may seem like the Child Archetype represents the notion of play, and in essence it does. But it isn't until the Child Archetype shifts into a communication style of acceptance, love, joy, and peace that it can play without an agenda and with no strings attached. Real, unfettered play is essential to life! It allows us truly to put our worries away and refill our emotional "storage tank." It isn't until the Child Archetype emotionally evolves that true joy can be experienced!

When I'm feeling most stressed, I know this is the time to step away from my struggles and challenges—even just my racing thoughts—and do something that has nothing to do with accomplishment, achievement, or responsibility. I know it's time to play!

For me, play is everything from listening to music and dancing around my family room, while my husband plays his drums or guitar; to sitting by a bonfire and gazing at the stars (which we do many nights during the summer months); to having a picnic lunch down at the lake with my kids and dogs.

Play is anything that brings you joy and pleasure! It's what fills you up and resets your Emotional Edge! Whether it's doing something physical such as playing sports, golfing, or dancing; something artistic like painting, writing, or sculpting; or anything else that brings you joy, excitement, and pleasure, play expands your Emotional Edges! It's not something that you should do only when you feel really burned out, or as a rare treat every once in a long while; Brown says that play "is vital for problem solving, creativity, and relationships."

The saying "All work and no play makes Jack a dull boy" is 100 percent true. If you don't balance your stress with more fun you will overload and burn out—no matter who you are or how strong and smart you feel. The most empowered and successful people know this secret!

Brown has spent decades studying the potency of play in everyone from prisoners to businesspeople to artists to Nobel Prize winners. He's reviewed more than six thousand "play histories," or case studies, that explore the role of play in each person's childhood and adulthood. For instance, he found that a lack of play was just as crucial as other influences in predicting criminal behavior among murderers in Texas prisons. He also observed that playing together helped couples revitalize their relationship and enhance emotional intimacy.

Similarly to how we arrange "playdates" for our children, I urge you to create your own "playdate" weekly! And if you're in an intimate relationship (especially one that is struggling), take the pressure off of having long, serious talks or strategy sessions for getting through the week. Instead, go do something fun together—something to engage both of you in an activity that allows you to be "present"—mindful. This may be the best marital advice you'll ever get!

Let go of the monkey business going on in your brain and let your heart and soul be refilled with some good old-fashioned fun! With a new, lighter perspective, everything in your life will look a little brighter!

## SMELL THE ROSES

I don't know anyone who doesn't feel calmer, happier, and more at peace after they've spent time in nature. In fact, "green therapy," also known as "ecotherapy," is gaining the attention of researchers in its ability to alleviate symptoms of depression.

A recent study conducted by scientists at the University of Essex found that taking a walk in nature reduced depression scores in 71 percent of participants. Researchers compared the effect with a control group who also took a walk, but in a shopping center. Only 45 percent of the shopping center walkers had reduced depression scores, while 22 percent of them actually felt more depressed.

Being in nature has been proven to improve mental health, boost self-esteem, help people with mental health problems return to work, improve physical health, and reduce social isolation.

I know for me the difference between walking on my treadmill and pounding the pavement outside is dramatic: after running outside I feel much more rejuvenated, inspired, and energized. (Although exercising inside will still noticeably improve my mood compared with not exercising at all!)

There is nothing like fresh air for clearing out the cobwebs and helping to reset your emotional baseline! As American author Richard Louv says in his book *The Nature Principle*, people living in high-tech societies often suffer from what he calls "nature deficit disorder." He insists:

> By tapping into the restorative powers of nature, we can boost mental acuity and creativity; promote health and wellness; build smarter and more sustainable businesses, communities, and economies; and ultimately strengthen human bonds.

In my own life, the most dramatic shift that occurred to me as an adult was in February 1997, when I decided to get my butt up every morning at six a.m. to head outside (first to go for a walk, and then later to jog). This single act of combining exercise with nature was the catalyst that allowed me to begin to step into my power and become the Adult Archetype.

As the years went on, I would fall off the wagon and then climb back on, but nothing has proven more impactful on my emotional well-being and, ultimately my business and my life's purpose, than exercising in nature.

Get outside, my friend, and let Mother Nature sprinkle her love down upon you.

## Your Sacred Space

Your outer world is a reflection of your inner world. It is *not* a reflection of who you *really* are, but it does reveal the Dominant Energy you've been in.

Just like your diet isn't going to change everything about your life, you can't simply clean up your outer world and expect all your problems to be solved. Your outer world is "effect." Your inner world is "cause." Until you get to the root of the problem, your outer world will continue to present you with unwanted results. It will show you the messages, thoughts, and beliefs of your inner world.

Take a look at your outer world, beginning with your home. Is it beautiful, clean, warm, loving, cozy, and inviting? Or is it disorganized, chaotic, overwhelming, and messy?

Don't get caught up in guilt or blame here. Just become the observer. Be a fly on the wall and simply observe the truth. Your home is an indication of where you're at emotionally. It reflects how you feel about yourself and your life.

Your home should be your safe haven, and within it, you need to have a Sacred Space where you can go to write, reflect, meditate, and pray. If you don't have a Sacred Space now, it's time to create one!

Sayings such as "cleanliness is next to godliness" have stood the test of time for a reason. We all feel better living in a clean, warm, loving home. Now, I'm not suggesting that your place should feel like a mausoleum or look like a model home. When

I spend time in houses that are so perfect they don't feel lived in, I can't help but wonder if their owners feel just as disconnected in their inner world. Warm, organized, and cozy homes are different from immaculate, controlled, and cold spaces. My own Sacred Space is a small bedroom I converted into my office and meditation room. With beautiful organza material and a staple gun, I turned the ceiling into a magical-looking tent, similar to what you'd see in a harem. I replaced the ceiling light with a chandelier and a dimmer switch, then added big pillows, plants, flowers, candles, crosses, statues, and lovely music. When I enter my office, I instantly feel better. When I feel better, I am more closely aligned with my Self. I get into the flow easier.

Room by room, I have created this feeling of love, safety, and security in my entire home—inside and out. I urge you to do the same.

Your Sacred Space doesn't need to be a whole room (especially if your place is small). It can be just a corner where you can put a rocking chair (or something comfy to sit on), along with a side table for your journal, pen, candle, flowers, and whatever else creates a sense of the sacred for you, including religious statues, books, a rosary or mala beads, and so on.

In time, you can slowly tackle your entire home so that your entire safe haven is reflecting back to you love, light, serenity, peace, joy, beauty, and sensuality. One step at a time! Have the patience to do what you can, without allowing yourself to become overwhelmed by the bigger picture.

If your Sacred Space is in your office, be sure to clean up your desk and light some candles to create the positive energy that will allow you to feel clear, appreciated, important, and worthy. You must make a separation between work time and rejuvenation time. This will also begin to shift your emotions around work and money. Your office needs to be a place you enjoy being in, especially if you plan on being financially independent and prosperous.

If your Sacred Space is in your bedroom, the same thing applies. Clean up your clothes (even give away any of your wardrobe that doesn't reflect the Real You!).

Make your bed every morning and get yourself some beautiful new sheets! Get rid of any junk, light some candles, and turn your room into your love nest. If you're single and looking for love . . . or married and trying to get pregnant . . . this is especially important for you to do as soon as possible.

Finally, it's important that there be no television in your Sacred Space. If it's absolutely impossible to remove it, though, be sure it's *not turned on* while you're reading this book, meditating, or journaling. There should be no distractions and/or low-resonating sources of energy in your Sacred Space.

You'll soon discover this journey is sacred because you are sacred. You must begin to create a Sacred Space that is worthy of the person you really are.

I've been coaching people for over twenty years, and I guarantee you this: when I ask them, months or even years later, what process was the most memorable of all the tasks I gave them—creating a Sacred Space is inevitably in the top two or three, every time.

Coming home is a metaphor for coming home to your Self!

Having a home that represents you—your creativity, beauty, passions, joys—is imperative to keeping this sacred journey alive. Without fail, those who live in a clean, organized, pretty place are more apt to keep their thoughts positive and their energy high.

Don't underestimate the power of your Sacred Space!

◼

Now that you have tackled my seven techniques for creating connection within your physical self, you will begin to feel strong enough to transcend to a higher energy. Keep practicing these techniques, even when it gets hard and you feel frustrated. Keep striving to do a little more, feel a little more, own a little more.

As you do this, get ready to take the next step with me, which is to begin to examine all of your relationships and the lessons they have to teach you.

# CHAPTER SEVEN

# Who Are You?

## "EMBRACE"

If you really want peace in the world, create peace in
your heart, in your being.
That is the right place to begin with and then spread.

OSHO

The first three-quarters of this book have been focused on
ourselves for a reason: everything in our outer world is a reflection of our inner world.

Our relationships are a reflection of ourselves. Our health,
income, and sex lives are also a reflection of how we are showing up in the world—how expansive or contracted we are.

We can't and won't see anyone else clearly—as *they* really
are—until our own lenses are clear and our perspective or context is empowered. Everything is relevant. Until we ourselves

are healthy in body, mind, and spirit, our relationships can't be healthy; and we can't create and sustain success, happiness, and love. We must be self-possessed before we can even think about influencing change in the outer world.

Your relationship can be only as healthy as the unhealthiest part of you.

If we had spent the majority of this book focused on our outer world—without healing the underlying cause of those choices—we'd simply redirect our wounds and suffering into a different manifestation. Sure, one aspect of our lives would perhaps improve, but something else would worsen.

Think about it: How many times have you seen the quiet, meek, heavy woman lose weight only to become a skinny, self-sabotaging, life-of-the-party girl still desperately seeking approval? Or the gangly kid who starts working out, puts on tons of muscle, and becomes a callous playboy—the Charmer? I'm sure you've witnessed the Narcissist or the Warrior who, after suffering a few traumatic setbacks, becomes the Addict, the Victim, or the Lone Wolf?

*If not addressed, one fear simply redirects into another form of self-sabotage.*

My philosophy has always been simple: focus on the inside and the outside will transform on its own. This is how long-term success is sustained.

Now don't get me wrong: you can't sit cross-legged in the lotus position and meditate all day or spend your waking hours journaling, reading, praying, and processing and expect your life to improve. You have to live in this world, experience others, engage in relationships, communicate and advocate, and develop deep and lasting connections, which is why this chapter is changing our focus from looking inward to looking outward!

We're going to begin to pay attention to how we are showing up in all our relationships and how those relationships either serve us or hurt us.

Let's start with our love lives . . .

## Men and Women

One of the easiest ways to recognize our Emotional Age is
through our relationships—especially our most intimate ones.
If we are resonating in love, our personal relationships are loving. If we are resonating in anger, our personal relationships
are angry. If we feel like an exhausted parent or a wounded
child, *we probably are.*

But on an even greater, more collective, historical level,
we've never experienced a world that allowed for empowered
women, until now—and that is only in most of the industrial-
ized, Western countries.

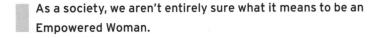

**As a society, we aren't entirely sure what it means to be an
Empowered Woman.**

In the Introduction, I wrote that this book is, in part, an
attempt to define what being an Empowered Woman means,
*and the answer to this will serve men, too!* Before we can have loving, intimate, empowered "love relationships," we must understand what has happened and is still happening to women
and, ultimately, to men because of women—*especially in the last
fifty years.*

I think we can all agree that men and women have never
before tried to navigate their relationships and love lives
under the drastically changing atmosphere that has permeated
Western society in the last century. Once we understand this

phenomenon, we will better understand how we need to navigate in love.

In order for us to continue to expand our relationships into the beautiful, loving places that we so badly want and need, we must learn how to communicate in a way that empowers both us and our partners. We need to create a new Love Language.

As the Dalia Lama said, it will be women who heal the world, and this means our turning toward our partners with compassion, empathy, understanding, and a desire to elevate them.

At this stage in history, it is important for women to realize that we need to treat one another the way that we want, deserve, and demand to be treated. We need to show men *who we really are*—not the constricted, fearful, angry versions of ourselves or the coy, cute damsel in distress.

For all the same reasons that women are in a period of enormous change, so, too, are men. As women's roles have changed so radically, in that we really don't have role models or blueprints to follow, men are experiencing the same thing. Not to mention, so-called patriarchal countries are watching those of us in the Western world, looking to see if "giving women power" will pay off in the long run.

When women collectively rise up and through the disempowerment that has permeated our gender for thousands of years, all of our lives will improve. We will feel expansive rather than restricted.

When women stop navigating their lives from passive or passive-aggressive archetypes, and when men start seeing women through the eyes of equality, dignity, and reverence, the world as a whole, including our love lives, will shift into a more empowered, accepting, loving place.

Men have always had the right to pursue their dreams,

build careers without feeling guilty, have children without losing themselves, and still feel entitled to make love at the end
of the day! Women are learning this now—for the first time
in history. As we become more empowered, we will be better
partners, not worse! Better mothers! Better negotiators! Better
communicators! Better entrepreneurs! Teachers! Leaders! Better! Happier!

Anger will diminish as we stop blaming and "hating" men!
Equality will flourish. Families will regain their footings. This
is a good thing! But it's up to us women to take the lead in
creating a new Love Language.

## THE TRUTH, THE WHOLE TRUTH, AND NOTHING BUT THE TRUTH

Many of us forget what life was like for our great-grandmothers.
Although our great-grandmothers didn't shoulder the burden
of making money or paying the bills, their future and that of
their offspring depended entirely upon the men they married. These women prayed the men in their lives would be
gentle and loving because if they weren't, the women had no
recourse. They prayed their men would be good providers and
would bring home their weekly paychecks: if the men didn't,
the women *couldn't*.

During the early history of the United States, men owned
their wives and children. Women couldn't keep their names
or possess any assets—even their inherited family homes became the property of their husbands. If men chose to send their
children to an orphanage, the mothers had no defense. The
women also had no rights over their own bodies, although *the
men* had full rights over their wives' bodies.

Crimes against women weren't considered serious. Although

women's "purity" was expected, rape was almost impossible to prove, and unless a black man faced charges for raping a white woman, the punishment was negligible. Women simply weren't deemed valuable—at least, not in the eyes of the law. You can imagine the rage women must have felt. It's no wonder that when feminism came along, women chose to fight for their rights and to stand up for themselves.

And where did all this leave us?

*Reeling in the aftermath . . .*

Men had no idea what to do, what to say, or how to emotionally support their wives. *(And most still don't!)* Some men truly don't even understand what women are so upset about: *"Can't you just get dinner ready and we'll talk about this later, honey?"*

It was the battle of the sexes—a war was waged, and we all woke up to the aftermath of destruction.

The women's movement had unleashed a tropical storm that left men feeling bruised, beaten, and totally and utterly confused. It left them no longer feeling "needed or respected"—*the very worst things that can happen to a man's ego.*

These men were our fathers, brothers, sons, and husbands. Most of these men did indeed need a good scolding (and millions still do). But many others just wanted to come home to a happy wife, a happy life, and a secure future; they wanted to pick up the pieces and rebuild: *"Tell me what to do and I'll do it!"*

## Love, Sweet Love

So how can we put down our weapons and begin the peace negotiations in earnest? In this section, I want to talk about living in a place of love that radiates out to your most important relationships.

Let's be honest: there are few things better in life than being in love! We are not meant to be solitary creatures. We are meant to share our hearts and have fulfilling, full-time, mutually satisfying relationships with individuals who, in turn, share their love with us.

But let's look at what happens to most of us: In the Western world, dating might go something like this:

When a woman first meets a guy and they start dating, she loves when he acts like a "man." She loves that he wants her! She loves that *he wants* to think up ways to make her happy. Nothing feels better than being adored by him! She laughs at his jokes and thinks he's so cute! But innately she knows that she needs to play a little hard to get. He is the hunter. He feels alive trying to win her! She feels alive being chased! He needs to show her he can provide, protect, be a good mate, and possibly even be the future father to her children (depending on their age and status in life). He'll be her knight in shining armor, if she'll let him.

And so *she* invites him over—legs shaved, roast in the oven, candles lit. She knows exactly how to seduce him! She'll be his everything! Actually, she *becomes* his everything!

*"Sure, baby! I don't mind. I'll do that for you. I'll do anything for you!"*

And he would do anything for her! An honest man will tell you that when he falls for a woman, he falls "hook, line, and sinker!" He'll jump hoops to please her!

When a man loves, he loves fiercely. When he commits, he brings all of himself to his relationship. If you treat him well, he's in it for life. Ever heard the Percy Sledge song "When a Man Loves a Woman"?

*She can do no wrong!*

(Let's tell the truth, ladies: this has been the strategy for thousands of years. "There are two ways to a man's heart," we've been told, "good food and good sex.")

Then, once she's got him, *she* changes!

She starts out cooking *all* the meals, doing his laundry, and picking up his socks (just like his mother did). She grumbles and complains. She starts telling him how to dress, how to do his hair, maybe even how to floss his teeth. She may begin making fun of the little silly things he has *always* done. (For God's sake, I've heard women complain about the way their man breathes.)

*We're only trying to help him improve. What's the problem?*

Or maybe the reverse: She stops taking care of him the way he's become accustomed to relying on her to do. Instead of homemade meals, she grabs takeout or defrosts whatever's in the freezer. She throws on the mismatched cotton undies that used to get saved for laundry day instead of the matching lingerie she used to choose carefully for him. She stops laughing at all of his jokes, stops shaving her legs, then becomes furious with him if he dares to mention any of these changes.

Our collective female consciousness is both angry and yet still needy, although much of the time we aren't even entirely sure what we're so mad about. Not to mention, we don't need men anymore! *And we let them know it!*

No matter! She starts telling her girlfriends, mother, and sisters (or *anyone* who is willing to listen) how much he's changed. He's not there for her anymore. Should she leave him? Should she stay? Or should she just keep complaining?

The power struggle is on. The relationship is doomed!

*He* starts shutting down. He's afraid that no matter what he does, it won't be good enough. So he retreats to his man cave:

his garage, basement, or local pub. She gets angry; what happened to her man? So she starts shutting down, too, without realizing that *she is part of this*!

## LADIES, WAKE UP!

One of the hardest lessons I've had to learn, and what I believe most women have a very challenging time with (especially after they have children) is learning the art of receiving—receiving pleasure, help, compliments, money, attention, support, even gifts, you name it. Many women have forgotten about this most feminine aspect of being a woman!

You may not even be sure what I mean by "receiving." The Merriam–Webster's Dictionary defines *receiving* as:

: to get or be given (something)
: to react to (something) in a specified way
: to welcome (someone) in usually a formal way

Without trying to be inappropriate, let's compare men and women in relationships to the sexual act:

Men are designed to "give";
Women are designed to "receive."

In day-to-day life, men are designed to give. They still want and *need* to provide, protect, and serve. They want desperately to be needed. It is part of their masculine hardwiring. If they can protect and serve, their testosterone soars. But when a man no longer feels needed, he feels worthless. His self-esteem plummets. Marriage Breakdown 101.

Women who navigate their relationships—particularly

their love lives—from the Parent Archetype can inadvertently emasculate their partners because they are always behaving like the primary giver and rarely like the receiver.

## TRANSCENDING THE PARENT

For those of you who struggle in the Parent Archetype, it is important to relax and try to let go of the reins a little! In heterosexual relationships, this means women must stop mothering their men and focus more on self-care and self-love, *and allow men to do the giving.* Of course, this goes against thousands of years of women being told that they should put their own needs last and the needs of their family's first.

Yes, you will always honor your sense of responsibility and trustworthiness, but unless you start to have more fun and adopt a less self-righteous and nagging style, if you do meet someone who is empowered, eventually, one of four things will occur:

1. The Adult will move on (this relationship is too oppressive). You are not their parent, and an empowered Adult will not stand to be treated like a child.
2. The Adult will start acting like the child and you like the parent. You'll find yourself in a codependent relationship. (And there's a good chance he'll cheat on or betray you.)
3. The Adult will turn into the parent. (If you can't beat them, join them!) You'll both soon feel bored and, perhaps, undesirable, but no one is going anywhere. This relationship may last, but your sex life will suffer dramatically, as your needs and desires are squelched.
4. You will let your hair down and start acting like the Adult and the relationship will blossom!

If you want this relationship to soar, your life has to become about you again—not the patterns that you've fallen into, and not even the person you aspire to be but have not yet attained, but the real *you*! If not, you'll continue to focus your frustrations and energy on what your partner is or isn't doing to make you happy.

Earlier in this book, I encouraged you to focus on your Self! Focus on your joy. Heal your heart. Have more fun and less seriousness. Take care of your needs. Protect yourself and your interests. You matter! This is the most important thing you can do to improve your love life.

Striving to grow and to heal can be a lifelong process. But as you turn toward your partner, think about how you can provide the kind of loving support that you yourself crave.

> The secret for women to remember is to always maintain a little "thrill of the chase," along with a gentle stroke of her man's ego!

Yes, keep your edge! Keep your opinions, friends, hobbies, interests, and desires. I know this may ruffle some feathers, but I actually believe it is important for the man to love the woman more. (Or at least, he must believe he does!) Don't lose yourself in the relationship by becoming too available and too focused on what your partner needs—even after years of marriage. You have to show him love and respect, but don't be googly-eyed and passive. Be his partner. His lover. His friend. His companion. His future.

On the other hand, don't let him get away with being disrespectful toward you. Be an empowered woman but not his mother! It's the only way to enable him to be an empowered man who will want to love, protect, and take care of you for a lifetime! Make a commitment to stop doing for him and giving so much to him. Stop asking him how he is, how he feels, what he needs, if he's hungry, or what's wrong?

It may sound as though I'm asking you to be a tad rude, but I'm not; I'm simply requesting that you stop acting like his mother or caretaker. You don't need to manage his moods, emotions, diet, or finances. You don't tell him how to eat, what to eat, how much to eat, or anything else regarding his diet . . . or *his drinking, for that matter*! You can provide healthy meals, when it's your turn to cook. You can raise the bar for yourself nutritionally. You can exude great health and a sexy body. But you are not his parent, personal trainer, psychologist, or assistant. Besides, when he realizes that you are no longer nagging or babysitting him, you may be surprised at what happens!

Here are some final tips you can begin to practice right away if you're in the Parent Archetype:

- No more coddling, excusing, justifying, parenting, fixing, rescuing, or saving your partner. He or she is not your child.
- Don't respond the minute he texts or calls you. Don't be too available.
- Tell yourself something fabulous *about youself* every day.
- Buy yourself some pretty lingerie (no matter your size) and wear it.
- Stop using your shrill "mother" voice. This might mean taking your voice down a few octaves.
- Wear something soft and pretty to bed.
- Take a hot salt bath and light some candles (for yourself!).
- Put cream on your skin nightly.
- Take time out to exercise daily—even just a walk outdoors.
- Go online and buy yourself a vibrator (it will come in an inconspicuous parcel; no one will know what it is). Use it!

- Get your teeth whitened.
- Go for a bikini wax.
- Sign yourself up for some dance classes—belly dancing, pole dancing, ballroom dancing, even doing Zumba at your local health club is a riot.
- Dress more femininely.
- Watch a comedy and let yourself laugh. Really laugh!
- Have more fun.
- Have more sex.
- Trust in the bigger picture.
- Giggle.

I'm a huge believer in trusting our own inner wisdom. One way to listen to your heart is to ask questions similar to these:

- If I wanted to stop feeling like the Mother, I would _____ (fill in the blank).
- If I wanted to feel like a Woman, I would _____ (fill in the blank).
- If I wanted a beautiful relationship, I would _____ (fill in the blank).
- If I wanted to be a better partner, I would _____ (fill in the blank).
- (For heterosexual women): If I wanted to help him feel like my Man, I would _____ (fill in the blank).

## TRANSCENDING THE CHILD

For those of you who struggle in the Child Archetype, it is important that you grow up! Yes, you always want to keep your youthful energy and maintain the part of you that is fun and playful, but unless you start acting like an empowered adult, if you do meet someone who is perfect for you, eventually, one of four things will occur:

**1.** The Adult will move on (this relationship is too toxic).

**2.** The Adult will start acting like the child (if you can't beat them, join them). This relationship will initially be fireworks but will soon become dangerous and unhealthy.

**3.** The Adult will turn into the Parent (overly protective and exhausted). You'll soon feel controlled and oppressed, like a child.

**4.** You will grow up and start acting like the Adult, and the relationship will blossom!

Unless you take action to stop the drama, dysfunction, temper tantrums, mood swings, addictions, commitment issues, and/or cheating, your relationships won't work. You are too intense. Too extreme. Too unhealthy.

If you have been navigating your relationship (or hoping to get into a relationship) as the Child, I'm here to tell you that no matter who you end up with, unless you start thinking "we" instead of "me," no relationship will ever fulfill you for the long term. You'll never find your bliss. Manipulation or passive-aggressive ploys will never empower you or bring you a soul mate love affair. Set fair and healthy boundaries; keep your sense of Self; don't let your partner be the only thing in your world, but don't become a diva, either!

Remember, loving your partner is giving him what he needs, as much as expecting him to meet your needs. Our relationships thrive when we walk that fine line—a balancing act of selflessness and selfishness!

Here are some final tips that you can begin to practice right away if you're in the Child Archetype:

■ No more ultimatums.

■ No more baby talk.

- No more competing or comparing.
- No more self-punishment.
- No more plastic surgery.
- No more whining.
- No more weighing yourself.
- No more adding drama to your stories.
- No more lashing out and misdirecting your frustrations.
- No more complaining.
- No more gossiping or snooping.
- No more sending angry text messages (especially after ten p.m.!).
- No more talking negatively about yourself—your body, personality, intelligence, or future.
- No more dwelling in the past.
- No more cutting up men (or other women, for that matter).
- No more spending money you don't have.
- No more using your sexuality to get your way.
- Look within; the answers are there.

## FINAL TIP, GALS

Here's the truth only a few of us have learned: no one is coming to save us! Nobody can change our lives, or nobody can help us with a problem that we haven't already accepted the responsibility for.

The good news: we women are finally saving ourselves! And this is important for global consciousness! We are learning how to expand the Emotional Edges of our universe—our horizon line of possibilities!

The empowerment of women is crucial for the expansion of consciousness. It is crucial in order to achieve world peace that the bonds between men and women blossom—and expand together!

When it comes to relationships, women must remember that no one can take our emotional power from us; only we can give it away. In fact, the power we naturally possess over men is so great, we must learn to wield it properly and responsibly.

One of the best things that women can do is to let the atmosphere in our relationships lift and lighten. I know it may feel counterproductive, but *stop talking* about your problems with the person who seems to be at the root of them; you're angry and need to express yourself! But let's not kid ourselves: there is nothing new to be gained by arguing. Focus on making your Self and your own life happier. Focus on Radical Self-Love and watch every aspect of your life—including your relationship—improve!

Once your partner feels this subtle yet significant change, he'll be open and willing to help more, show you more affection, and yes . . . have those long talks that you desire!

The reason for this is because when men are in the heat of battle, the last thing they want to do is talk. They are designed to protect and serve. It's as though they're down in the trenches and the bullets are flying and they're trying to stay alive . . . *and you want to talk*. When things start lightening up and the pressure isn't so tense, even a normally quiet man will feel relaxed enough to join your conversations.

I get that we women must talk about our troubles! Our bodies release a feel-good hormone called oxytocin when we chat and share our struggles. This hormone buffers the fight-or-flight response and counters stress, while producing a calming effect. *But it works in the reverse for men.* Unlike women, men have *only* a fight-or-flight response to stress. Talking about their problems lowers their feel-good hormone, testosterone. It diminishes their happiness. It drains them. They want to flee . . . from us . . . fast!

If you've ever gone to marriage counseling, how many times have you left the therapist's office only to find that you and your partner are in a bigger mess than when you arrived? Your man is miserable even though you felt better talking it out! But now you're in an argument because he is stonewalling you.

Researchers at UCLA found the following:

> Women have a larger behavioral repertoire than just fight or flight, when the hormone oxytocin is released as part of the stress responses in a woman. This calming response does not occur in men because testosterone—which men produce in high levels when they're under stress—seems to reduce the effects of oxytocin. Estrogen seems to enhance it.

If you've ever seen guys get together for a beer after work, very rarely will you hear them talking about their relationship problems. They want to escape their worries. They want to feel better and focus on things that lift their spirits. They talk about sports, music, politics, investments, cars, renovations, the weather, even the hot girl at the office—anything other than their problems. Women call this "sweeping things under the carpet." Men may disagree.

Now, I don't mean to suggest that we shouldn't communicate our problems and needs with our partners because they don't want to hear us complain. Not at all! But once we are clearer about how we are showing up in our relationship and what this is really all about, we can communicate with our partners in a much healthier way than most of us have been doing—without the blame, shame, or judgment.

I know in my marriage, my husband desperately struggled when I was unhappy and yet he was unable to talk with me

about my unhappiness. This fear of facing our problems together often created conditions for the perfect storm. I needed
to express myself but he was afraid to give me the space I
needed: *What if talking turned into arguing? What if validating my
emotions escalated them and I became depressed?* In his mind, better
to not "go there" at all.

I felt stonewalled. Ignored. Neglected. I would criticize
him for his inability to communicate about anything except
"good" things. He'd become defensive and shut down. It was
a vicious cycle.

I finally understood that my husband "took on" my pain
and became upset with *himself* when he couldn't "fix" me.
Sadly, it translated to me that I couldn't ever show my unhappiness and that if I did, it meant I was "broken."

Once I realized this was my story—that is, *"I suffer in silence.
No one really cares about my needs"*—and that he was merely mir-
roring it back to me, I was able to stop focusing on him and get
to work on myself! Remember: Our relationships are a reflection of our own beliefs.

Once my husband recognized that the deep sorrow I occasionally felt wasn't really about him and his shortcomings,
and that I wasn't holding him responsible for my lifetime of
letdowns, and that I simply needed him to listen without fixing, rescuing, or even lecturing me, he was willing to give me
what I needed: validation, love, and compassion. Our relationship began to blossom in a whole new way!

Truth be told, once I was willing to give myself what I
needed—validation, love, and compassion—I was able to receive it from my husband.

When we can be honest with our partner about those indelible marks that have changed the trajectory of our lives, we
can help them better understand our vulnerabilities and why

we are showing up as a particular Emotional Sub-Archetype. We stop blaming and start healing. We stop arguing and start listening.

It is also interesting to note that women's brains have evolved differently than men's over time. We have thousands of connective tissues linking the right and left hemispheres of our brain, something that men don't have. This means, in a sense, we can open up different drawers in our "mental" filing cabinet and access all of them, all at the same time. I think most men will admit they become overwhelmed listening to a group of women chatting—hence the term *henhouse*. We women can carry on ten different conversations all at once and never lose track of what we are talking about.

Men, on the other hand, use one side of their brain or the other, but never both simultaneously. They aren't wired to. Men need to focus on one thing at a time. Bombard a man with too much, and he'll shut down and become defensive. He'll stop talking. We call this stonewalling. We feel ignored and disrespected. Lonely. Unheard. Meanwhile, he feels flooded by our criticism and contempt.

According to marriage expert John Gottman, PhD, most marriages fail because of what he warns are "The Four Horsemen of the Apocalypse":

1. Criticism
2. Contempt
3. Defensiveness
4. Stonewalling

Here's my advice: Talk with your girlfriends. Talk with your mother, your coach, your therapist, pastor, priest, or any other trusted person who can offer you compassionate and supportive listening and wise advice. In fact, my international coaching school offers free empowerment coaching to any woman, living anywhere in the world: **www.SWATinstitute.com** (Simply Woman Accredited Trainer). There are no hidden catches or fees. We simply help you shift into a higher level of consciousness, which allows you to better communicate your needs and receive your partner's in an assertive, accepting, and loving way. As you both start to feel better, you'll be amazed at how easy it is to find resolutions to your problems—together.

## Guys, Listen Up!

Okay guys, you aren't off the hook!

Heterosexual men: you need to remember to treat your woman like a woman! Chivalry isn't dead! She wants you to wine, dine, and treat her fine! She doesn't want to be your mother or your daughter, nor do you want her to be!

*What guy wants to have sex with his mother, right?*

Even if you've been married for a while, it's important that you remember the little things that make her feel beautiful, feminine, and appreciated. So this means that, no matter whether you both agreed to "no gifts this Christmas," you still need to get her a little something; bring flowers home on your anniversary (or for no reason at all), give her perfume or chocolate on Valentine's Day; and give her something personal— *just for her*—on her birthday. This means no kitchen appliances or gadgets, no "us" gifts (things for the inside or outside of the house), or boring, comfy, mother-type presents. A lovely (even inexpensive) piece of jewelry goes a long way! A day at the spa is magnificent! Even just your own little coupons that offer a massage or back tickle! Remember the saying "Happy wife! Happy life!"

Become more mindful of yourself, your woman, and your relationship. Make the decision to really "be in it"! As my husband and I joke, "We're in it to win it!"

Think before you do things. Ask yourself:

"Will this upset her? Should I give her a quick call to tell her I'll be home late? What can I do this week to show her that I care? Am I helping enough around the house? How balanced is the workload? How happy am I? How can I ensure my woman knows how *desired and adored* she is by me? Am I doing the best job I can?"

You have to understand the enormous stress put on women in this day and age. John Gray, PhD, points out in *Venus on Fire, Mars on Ice*:

Almost 40 percent of women in America today are their family's primary breadwinner. Soon, the majority of workers in the U.S. may be women. That's unprecedented, and so is the amount of wealth that women control. What generations of women strove to accomplish—gaining more access to money and opportunity—seems to have been achieved. Yet, women face harder choices, greater unhappiness, and yes, higher levels of stress.

He goes on to explain:

When I talk about the enormous stress that women are experiencing today, some husbands living in America naively reply, "My wife isn't stressed; she's better off than 99 percent of the world's population!" This is a man who doesn't understand what stress really is. Basically, he's saying, "What does she have to complain about? We have a house and plenty of food in the refrigerator."

This attitude is just plain ignorant, and it can destroy a relationship. What such a man doesn't know or isn't accepting is that there are different kinds of stress. Poverty and the threat of starvation is one kind of stress. Living in a country with few opportunities for economic advancement is a different kind of stress. But, believe it or not, these kinds of stress are actually very low compared to the kinds of stress that men and women are experiencing in the modern world. Living life in a hurry while stuck in L.A. traffic can produce much higher levels of stress, as measured by cortisol levels, than living in a rural village with no electricity, no grocery stores, and little opportunity to live a better life.

When your woman feels less stressed, your life will become so much smoother and happier. She is responsible for her own happiness, but you can certainly change the atmosphere at home by helping out more and reducing her workload. When she is upset, practice listening without taking her feelings on as your own. You don't have to fix her but you do have to hear her. You will be shocked at how much gentler and more loving she'll be with you; she'll be far less nagging, and I guarantee that your sex life will get hotter! Good news for everyone!

Something else to keep in mind: the average forty-year-old man today has testosterone levels comparable to a seventy-year-old man from thirty years ago. Testosterone is a hormone. It's what puts hair on a man's chest. It's the force behind his sex drive. It's what makes him feel "manly"!

For a long time, doctors were not attributing many of the health concerns that men face today to low testosterone, but according to Jason Hedges, MD, PhD—a urologist at Oregon Health & Science University in Portland, "From diabetes, depression, high blood pressure, and coronary artery disease, low testosterone may be at the root of the problem."

If you feel like you're losing your mojo—if you're tired or depressed, have mood swings, a low sex drive, or erectile dysfunction (ED or impotence), see your doctor and ask for a blood test. Having blood work is the only way really to know how much testosterone you're producing.

If your levels are low, your doctor may prescribe testosterone. Here are the best ways for you to increase your testosterone naturally:

- Lose weight (overweight men have been proven to have less testosterone than fit men).
- Reduce your sugar intake (sugar is found in all processed foods; it inhibits the release of growth hormone, which is your feel-good, anti-aging, muscle-producing hormone).
- Engage in a twenty-minute, intense, interval cardio session daily (think sprinter versus long-distance runner).
- Lift weights three times a week—make sure the weights are heavy enough that you can do no more than six to ten repetitions (think strength versus endurance).
- Supplement your daily diet with at least 30 mg but no more than 40 mg of zinc.
- Get a short burst of sun daily—vitamin D (a steroid hormone) helps maintain semen quality and sperm count.
- Eat lean protein and healthy fats daily (healthy fats can be found in fish, nuts, avocado—guacamole—unheated olive oil, etc.).

I also encourage you to ask yourself similar questions— your own inner wisdom will guide you:

- If I wanted to stop feeling like her son (or her father), I would _____ (fill in the blank).
- If I wanted to feel like her man, I would _____ (fill in the blank).

- If I wanted to help her feel like my woman, I would _____ (fill in the blank).
- If I wanted a beautiful relationship, I would _____ (fill in the blank).
- If I wanted to be a better partner, I would _____ (fill in the blank).

And ladies, if your partner is unwilling to read this book or apply these suggestions, the next section outlines my tips *for you* to better get your needs met!

## Your Love Language

As I've mentioned already, you can't change something until you accept responsibility for it. If your needs are not being met, rather than sticking to the same old approach, why not try a new, more empowered strategy?

First things first, I'm assuming you're already operating *above* the level of Aggressive Communication and are, at the very least, navigating as the Assertive Adult Archetype. You've crossed the Assertiveness Bridge and are in the higher levels of consciousness.

If you are mindful of your relationship and you still find yourself unable to connect with your partner—truly and deeply—it is time for you to reach higher and expand your Emotional Edges for the sake of your Self, your relationship, your partner, and the collective consciousness!

So before you read on, it's important that you've already committed to operating as the Empowered Adult—to "fight fair," respect the other, and maintain your own self-respect.

If you haven't done these things, then you must go back to where you were and pick up the slack. Reread Chapters Three,

Four, and Five! You have some basic, fundamental changes you need to make before you'll be ready to shift into this more expansive communication style called Acceptance.

If you are ready to improve your relationship, the time has come for you to examine the slew of beliefs you've, most likely, unconsciously accepted along the way—the ones about judging, evaluating, and criticizing. These beliefs created your personal Love Language, which you bring into every relationship.

Until you reflect on what you've learned and discard the beliefs that aren't serving you, you will not be able to fully love and accept anyone—*especially yourself!*

It takes courage to be open-minded and accepting of people who are different than we are.

## WHAT IS A LOVE LANGUAGE?

Based on our own experiences, we have all internalized our own definitions of words and concepts. For example, what appears to be extreme devotion to one person may be inadequate attention to someone else. These beliefs form our Love Language.

Our Love Language is our interpretation of our beliefs about love, marriage, sex, intimacy, connection, care, sexiness, brawn, romanticism, male and female roles, and so on. These attitudes are subjective and relative, which is why there is no right way of looking at any of these concepts, but rather a perceived expectation.

In Chapter Two, I suggested that you look back at your earliest memories to see what you learned about love from your mother (if you're a woman) or from your dad (if you're a man). Your same-sex parent has had the biggest influence on your Emotional Age and how you're showing up in love.

You've made hidden commitments to be either just like Mom or just like Dad, or to be the complete opposite of one of them. You were locked into unconscious love patterns—living out the script you wrote many years ago—*long before you met your partner.*

As I already mentioned, patterns are nothing more than thoughts and beliefs passed down, generation after generation. If you want a beautiful, loving relationship, you have to change some of the unhealthy, limiting patterns.

If you learned that love is painful, dramatic, or dysfunctional, or that your love partner will eventually let you down, you will unconsciously create scenarios to affirm your beliefs. Your mind will twist reality in order to "see" your partner through these lenses.

Once you start to recognize the script that you've been following throughout your life, you can make changes in terms of how you are showing up in your relationship. The great news is this doesn't take therapy! Mindfulness and acceptance are needed most!

**Your relationship will be whatever you *believe* it will be.**

This calls to mind a story about my client, Dorian, that I shared in my book *Transcendent Beauty,* who was struggling in her fourth marriage and couldn't understand why she was attracting such selfish, cold, distant men when she was so loving and giving herself. After talking for about fifteen minutes, zeroing in on certain things she said, I asked Dorian if she was an only child. Surprised, she answered yes. I asked her to tell me what her beliefs were about being loved, and what life had been like for her while growing up.

My client responded that her parents doted on her, and

that her needs had always been met. To her, love meant that you shower the person you care about with lots of attention and affection.

"Mmm . . . what a wonderful childhood it seems you had," I pointed out. "So to you, being loved means being the center of attention. When people love you, they really need to show it to you through their actions, right?"

Dorian agreed that for her, being loved meant being absolutely adored and catered to in every way. She laughed as she said this, but then added, "But I give just as much attention as I demand!"

"I bet you do!" I smiled. "But how about your husband? What was his childhood like?"

"Oh . . . well, he had eleven siblings and a mother who worked nights as a nurse."

"Wow!" I exclaimed. "I wonder what 'love' means to him."

I could see that Dorian was getting it: beliefs aren't right or wrong; they're only perceptions of truth.

## WRITING YOUR NEW LOVE LANGUAGE

By learning what your own Love Language *has been up until now*, and then making the commitment to talk with your partner about both of your Love Languages—your current life scripts and Emotional Ages—you can explore your differences and similarities and determine what will allow you, as a couple, to create space for your new, mutually shared Love Language to blossom.

The power of language is huge. Simply stated: your choice of words and the context in which you express them deeply affects your relationships, probably in ways you don't even realize.

We have to be honest with ourselves about how we are

speaking, what we are saying, and the tone we are taking. Are we on the offense? Are we on the defense? Are we using a lot of absolute terms such as *never* and *always*? Are we open, loving, and positive—seeing things through good lenses or not so good lenses?

When we fall in love, we have to adjust ourselves and our view of things. We have to broaden our Love Language to meet both our and our partner's needs.

In countries with arranged marriages, the idea is about finding a partner for your child so the two share as many similarities as possible. These individuals believe that while opposites attract, "likes last."

The truth is, we don't have to come from the same religion or culture as our partner in order for us to be happy; however, we must have many similar values in order to sustain a healthy relationship. The secret is talking, sharing, and learning about each other, long before you tie the knot! And then keeping the lines of communication open! People change as they age. Our needs change.

*Some questions you can ask yourself (and your partner) while creating your own private Love Language are these:*

1. When you think of the word *love*, what immediately comes to mind?
2. Did you grow up seeing your parents in a loving, healthy relationship? What did you learn from them about love, intimacy, sex, commitment, etc.?
3. What Dominant Emotional Archetype were your parents in most often? How did that influence you?
4. Were your parents demonstrative and affectionate with each other in front of you (regardless of how they treated you or your siblings)? What did that teach you?

5. Did either of your parents cheat on the other? If so, how was that dealt with in your family?

6. Were you ever expected to play referee or to listen to either parent privately complaining about the other? If so, how did that affect you?

7. Do you trust easily? If not, is that a fair challenge for your current partner to face?

8. What Dominant Emotional Archetype has been showing up in your relationship? What Dominant Emotional Archetype has been showing up in your partner? How has this been working for you?

9. Are your romantic and sexual needs being met? If not, why do you believe that is?

10. What did your same-sex parent teach you about being sexually active?

11. Did you experience any trauma around sex? If so, how is that showing up in your love life today?

12. After learning about the different communication styles—from Passive to Peaceful—how did you most often see your parents communicating?

13. After learning about the different communication styles—from Passive to Peaceful—which way do you use most often to communicate with your partner?

14. How do you best like to show your partner that you love him or her?

15. How do you best like to be shown that you are loved?

16. What changes would you like to see your partner make for you?

17. What changes do you believe your partner would like to see you make for them?

18. Which of the above changes do you feel are possible? Why or why not?

**19.** Can you accept that your partner needs some help, time, and encouragement to make these changes?

**20.** Are you willing to share these answers with your partner and begin to create your own Love Language as a couple?

In the new book by Rob Bell and his wife, Kristin, called *The Zimzum of Love: A New Way of Understanding Marriage,* they write extensively about "holding space" for each other. They describe this space as something called *zimzum*:

There is a mysterious, indescribable, complex exchange that can happen in the space between you and your partner. You find each other. Your centers of gravity expand as your lives become more and more entwined. You create space for this other person to thrive while they're doing the same for you. This creates a flow of energy in the space between you. This energy field is at the heart of marriage.

This zimzum space is similar to what I was mentioning in Chapter Four, where I talked about loving each other so much you're willing to hold space for the relationship to blossom—and for your partner to expand his or her life. Acceptance, reason, and love are what you must turn toward to allow you to navigate together during tough times. Sometimes, in order to do this, we must forgive our partner for past mistakes.

Again, I stress: this is assuming you've already been negotiating and compromising in Assertive Communication or higher! If you aren't in the higher levels of consciousness, true forgiveness is impossible to achieve.

When we speak of Loving Communication, it ensures an enduring and unconditional promise in which we seek to include, express, and recontextualize negative feelings, emotions, beliefs, and situations into positive ones (and not just toward our partner but toward ourselves, as well). This means finding the "gift in the garbage" and then taking out the trash!

Just imagine if you or your partner is carrying around fifty pounds of past pain and suffering? The proverbial "elephant in the room" is with you at all times, even if you think you're hiding it well. This baggage is always intruding on your intimacy.

The saying "It is darkest just before dawn" gets to the essence of the Emotional Edge! This is the place where you consciously choose to let go of the anger you've been carrying for your well-learned lessons. You are wiser now. You've extracted the gifts. You know that it's time to let go of the rest. It's time to release the extra stuff. You're smarter, stronger, and more expansive. You jump! You let go! You soar! Relief rather than resistance is occurring! Expansion! Life! Love! Laughter! The Flow!

Besides, you've mastered the art of Empowered Communication, so if a healthy boundary needs to be maintained, you know now how to do it! You don't need to let yourself get angry or "even"—vindictiveness will destroy you! Instead, speak your needs in a "win-win" way, making sure that you are clear about the consequences, and then give love a chance. Hold space and trust that your partner will join you.

The great news is that once you forgive and wipe the slate clean, you'll be free to give yourself, your partner, and all who are close to you your beautiful love. And there's nothing better than the gift of love!

In Judaism on the High Holy Days, adherents grant forgiveness to anyone who has wronged them; they ask forgiveness of anyone whom they have wronged; and they ask forgiveness and release from G-d for any vows and oaths that they've sworn in the last year. I think this is a beautiful approach to which we should all look in our quest to become mindful of our need to forgive.

I believe that at least twice a year, say on Valentine's Day and on our anniversary (or some other significant date we share with our partner), we should sit for an hour or so of private reflection to atone for the ways in which we've judged, evaluated, and criticized our partner; then, we should look to see where we've fallen out of alignment with our mutual Love Language. We need to ask ourselves, "Where am I showing up self-righteously?"

It is also important to ask our partner's forgiveness for the mistakes we've made—knowingly or not. A simple prayer or request you may want to say is this:

> I pray that_____ (say the person's name) will have a good day, filled with love, compassion, and understanding. I ask that she/he will forgive me for _____ (fill in the blank, or simply refer to this as "whatever she/he believes I've done to hurt her/him"). I pray that I can forgive the ways she/he has hurt me, and that I will see her/him for who she/he really is. I pray she/he will see the Real Me, as well. I send you, _____ (say the person's name), love. Amen and amen.

You may need to say this prayer many days or weeks—even months—in a row in order to fully embody this loving state of being.

Once the slate is clean (and that first may mean some tears and/or even a physical break), stay mindful of *keeping the past behind you* and recommitting daily to your Love Language.

Speaking the same Love Language as your partner is paramount to your living a great life, filled with love, pleasure, and peace. But you need an accepting and loving heart to allow you to speak and listen, in a way in which both your needs are heard.

Understanding your partner's past Love Language doesn't mean you should accept poor treatment now because of what he or she has been through, but it does enable you to be more compassionate of his or her wounds, and to work together to write a new, mutually beneficial Love Language—one that works for both of you.

Gary Chapman, author of the bestselling book *The 5 Love Languages*, explains why most books and articles published about relationships miss out on this most fundamental truth: "People speak different love languages."

He believes there are five emotional love languages; in other words, five ways that we each speak and understand emotional love. They are through words of affirmation, quality time, receiving gifts, acts of service, and physical touch.

"Learning to speak the primary language of your spouse," he insists, "may radically affect his or her behaviour. People behave differently when their emotional love tanks are full."

Although I believe we have even more than five Love Languages (they are as unique as we are people), I agree that reflecting on what we learned while growing up about love, sex, intimacy, etc., and then sharing these insights with our partner is the first step to creating a new Love Language as a couple. We have to be willing to do our best to give our partner what they need emotionally, sexually, mentally, or physically in order to feel "full"—just as long as it doesn't compromise our personal integrity.

Empowered Communication encourages us to open up our hearts enough to be able to learn from our partner and to help expand our partner's life, which encourages us to expand our own life as well. This is what a healthy relationship looks and feels like. It brings out the best in us both.

This requires us to wake up and to be present—to expand our level of consciousness by paying attention to the "now" with all our senses. It requires us to unplug from the distractions and to become aware of "what is," where we both need to recontextualize our beliefs in order to give our partner the things we need in order to feel loved and respected. This is where selfishness and selflessness meet. We take joy in loving and pleasing our partner. It doesn't feel like sacrifice.

In *A New Earth*, spiritual mystic Eckhart Tolle shares:

> To be in alignment with "what is" means to be in a relationship of inner non-resistance with what happens. It means not to label it mentally as good or bad, but to let it be. Does this mean you can no longer take action to bring about change in your life? On the contrary. When the basis for your actions is inner alignment with the present moment, your actions become empowered by the intelligence of Life itself.

Intelligence is the force that flows through and around us, just as Gandhi spoke about. It is the Presence that Dr. David Hawkins described, "whose power is infinite, exquisitely gentle, yet rock-solid."

An empowered person—the Adult Archetype—is tapped into this Intelligent Presence. The Adult Archetype operates in the "now." Their sensuality—*or the awakening of all their senses*—is paramount to establishing happy, loving relationships. Being "present" is the secret sauce that makes love so spectacular! Joy arrives when we remain in this space with ease. Our love for our partner becomes "infinite, exquisitely gentle, yet rock-solid."

The bottom line, we can't be caught up in the past or wor-ried about the future; we must be "here and now," living each day to the fullest! Remember, suffering no longer serves us! We must set ourselves and our partner free! Forgive! And if new boundaries are needed, *set them*!

## WHEN IN DOUBT

The best advice I can give to both men and women is that *when in doubt, don't!*

Do not react when you feel upset—as challenging as I know this is! When you are feeling angry is not the time to interact. Step away! Don't get caught up in the moment. Grab ahold of yourself. Take a few deep breaths. Calm down. Let go. Manage your emotions. Overlook the obvious. Let it be. Let it be. Try to figure out what is really going on: *this* is rarely about *this*.

Your actions and reactions must improve or you'll keep get-ting the same results.

When in doubt, ask yourself, "What Dominant Emotional Archetype am I operating in? What archetype do I want to be operating in instead?"

Then imagine your greatest mentor or role model and again ask yourself: "What would she or he do in this situation?"

*If you can't find clarity with this simple approach, some other ques-tions you can ask yourself are these:*

1. What are my intentions?
2. What would I have to overlook or "let go of" in order to allow myself to shift to a higher emotional place?
3. Can I do this without compromising my integrity? If no, skip to Question 6.
4. Am I managing my emotions, or are they managing me?

5. Am I asking empowered questions, or am I focusing on the problem?
6. Is it time to negotiate new, healthier boundaries? If so, do I have the courage to have an assertive, yet compassionate "win-win" conversation?
7. If not, why not?

If, after asking yourself these seven questions, you still can't see beyond yourself and your side of the story, managing your emotions becomes your number one task.

This means you will have to learn how to pause, step away, and take the thirty-thousand-foot view to see things from both perspectives—yours and your partner's. This takes self-awareness and mindfulness, but mostly, it simply requires letting up on that fierce grip you have on life, on your partner, and most likely, on yourself.

There are few things better in life than love. Remember that!

## BETWEEN THE SHEETS

Let's be honest: sex is an important part of a healthy, happy, empowered relationship. It creates intimacy and connection, builds immunity to stress and illness, and solidifies an important aspect of life that only your sexual partner can bring to you. And to be bluntly honest: sex is the good stuff! The trouble is, for most people, a *healthy* sex life is the first thing to go when a person or a couple hits a rut.

The frustrating part for some couples is that a good sex life can't make a relationship but a bad one can certainly ruin it! And too many couples are being left unfulfilled by bad sex lives!

According to the book *Real Sex for Real Women* by Dr. Laura Berman,

> When you first met your lover, chances are you were overwhelmed with sensations of excitement, bliss, and smoldering desire. When you fall in love, your brain releases chemicals such as serotonin, adrenaline, and oxytocin. These chemicals create feelings of excitement and passion. As time goes by, and you become more comfortable together, your desire wanes and you stop having as much sex. This phase also tends to involve a loss of spark.
>
> This happens because, over time, your brain becomes accustomed to these chemicals and requires more hormones to create the initial high. In other words, ongoing intense sexual excitement in a loving relationship goes against our biological instincts. This means you have to work at keeping the intimacy and attraction between you.

I think the real trouble happens when we stop *being into ourselves*. I love the breakdown of the word *intimacy*—"in to me, I see."

When we stop taking care of ourselves, when we stop making our own health and happiness important, we lose our need and desire to connect intimately with our partners. We may want to blame them, but on some level we know we contributed to it.

I've always believed that our sex life is a great mirror that reveals to us how we are *really* showing up in the world. It's an inside look at which Dominant Emotional Archetype we truly embody.

If you've been resonating as the Parent for too long, you may feel nervous or uncomfortable reintroducing sexuality back into your relationship . . . even just with yourself. You may have been "closed-down for business." That's okay, and it's normal! Like the saying goes, "When we don't use it, we lose it!" The good news is that you can never lose your Self, and your sexuality is a part of your Self!

Make a list of all the qualities that a sexy, empowered adult would possess.

Find ways to start incorporating more sensuality (the awakening of all your senses) into your life, whether it's having a hot bath instead of a quick shower, taking time to put cream on your skin, and the most important one, getting to know your own body—what feels good, what pleasures you, what excites or stimulates you! One of the great ways I recommend rekindling things is to begin by reading a romantic novel that lights your inner fire. Notice the excitement you feel inside during the juicy parts! Yes, you are still alive!

Once you are more at ease with yourself, it will be much easier to be more at ease sexually with your partner!

If you've been navigating your life from the Child Archetype, you may have been using sex to get your own way or to avoid certain feelings. Just like the Parent Archetype, you have to get clear on what a healthy sex life looks and feels like to you. Maybe it's time you and your partner created a new, joint Love Language!

*Here are some additional ways to reinvigorate your sex life:*

- Take a look at your bedroom. Does it represent a space where intimacy and passion reside, or is it disorganized and messy, or alternatively, is it too sterile and cold? Commit to making your bedroom a haven of beauty, passion, and pleasure. Clean it up! Get it organized, light some candles, purchase a stereo to play romantic music, simmer different essential oils or sexy incense. And no pictures of your children or parents! In fact, if you have children, put a lock on your door for "Parent Private Time." This is your love nest!

- Simplify your obligations to others. Create the space in your life for relaxation, rejuvenation, and *pleasure*. If you're overwhelmed, sex is often the first place to suffer when more satisfying sex would help counterbalance all your stress!

- Commit to nonsexual but intimate activities with your partner every week: a back massage, foot rub, arm tickle, or even a bubble bath or shower taken together.

- Exercise or move your body at least three to four times a week. Movement makes you feel younger, sexier, and more confident. It dramatically helps with "keeping Your mojo!"

- Go out by yourself or with same-sex friends more often. A *little* absence makes the heart grow fonder, but too much can create too much distance. Let your partner miss you but not forget you!

- Create a list of the most intimate memories you've ever had with your lover, and every so often send an e-mail reliving it—detail for detail! Both of your sexual neurons will be firing off excitement. This is awesome foreplay!

- Never compare your body to your younger years (or to someone else's body). No matter your clothing size, you deserve to be adored and pleasured!

- Learn how to pleasure yourself, and do it often! One of the secrets to increased intimacy is learning to please yourself! Let your own brain create your wildest fantasies about you and your partner! You are training your brain to become more sexual! If you feel courageous, share your honest desires with him or her! I guarantee it will reignite the passion between you, and you'll gain such a sense of sexual freedom!

■ Thoughts become things: become mindful about having sex, feeling sexy, and making sex a priority.

■ Practice being sexy. Ask yourself, "If I felt sexier, I would _____ (fill in the blank)." *Then, do it!*

■ No matter how long you and your partner have been to-gether, go out on a *first* date (often): laugh, have fun, and flirt. Eat with good manners. Show interest. Turn off your phone, and do not check it even once during dinner. Unplug from all the distractions that put distance between you and your mate. Plug back into him or her. Your partner will love it! And you'll love how he or she reciprocates that love! Keep reminding yourself over the course of the evening: "This is our first date!" If things should progress to the bedroom, make love like it's your first time, too. Things are guaranteed to stay fresh forever!

Love heals everything, and a great sex life is the topping on the cake! Decide that you matter! Sex matters! And your partner's pleasure matters!

One thing that can be incredibly hard on a relationship is the struggle to get pregnant. Then, what should be the most intimate and joyful act between a couple can become bur-densome and emotionally painful. My best advice to you, if you're in that situation, is to forget about sperm and egg unit-ing. Focus on falling in love and having fun again! Focus on feeling good again! Intimacy is the ultimate creation. And to be honest, if the woman isn't enjoying herself—if she does not orgasm during the act of making love—her body is simply not as relaxed and receiving of his body. Both people must win for it to be empowered!

# CHAPTER EIGHT

# What's My Purpose?

## "SOAR"

> Everybody is a genius. But if you judge a fish by its
> ability to climb a tree,
> it will live its whole life believing that it is stupid.
>
> ALBERT EINSTEIN

## Follow Your Bliss

*"What's my purpose?"*

Isn't this the "million-dollar" question that so many of us ask?

We live in an ever-expanding, infinite universe. We're made of the same stardust that the planets are made of. It stands to reason that we are a microcosm of the whole and our purpose here on Earth is for each of us to live our lives in full expansion; to trust, try, and believe in our dreams; to go for it all; and live a larger-than-life experience.

Our purpose is to expand—not just extend—our lives! And the good news is that since we are "infinite," we can relax about the "extension" part.

> When you live your greatest life, not only does your life expand, collective consciousness expands.

Sadly, too few of us were taught "I can trust life. I can trust myself. I can follow my bliss. I can dream—*big!*"

Maybe you learned that life is hard, that what goes up must come down, and that bliss is a fleeting moment that passes as quickly as a beautiful sunset.

Some of us are afraid that we have to enjoy our success while it lasts because it is limited and short-lived. Others believe that we have to force, demand, manipulate, or exhaust ourselves in the pursuit of happiness; that we'll be rewarded only if we work hard enough for someone else to notice.

Perhaps you've come to believe that if you can just persevere long enough, good things will be waiting on the other side of suffering. For some people, this means living a life of misery in order to get into heaven. For others, it means taking the safe path with plan B without ever testing out plan A. And for still others, it means listening to an internal voice that says, "Play it safe. Play it small. Don't take any leaps. Get back from the edge!"

In this mind-set, you struggle with sadness, discomfort, suffering, sorrow, guilt, shame, regret, blame, anger, illnesses, exhaustion, and/or addictions, convinced that it is part and parcel to discovering happiness. It is not true. Happiness won't arrive at the end of an unhappy life.

Shawn Achor, author of *The Happiness Advantage*, is one of the world's leading experts on human potential. His work reveals:

> More than a decade of groundbreaking research in the fields of positive psychology and neuroscience has proven in no uncertain terms that the relationship between success and happiness works the other way around. Thanks to this cutting-edge science, we now know that happiness is the precursor to success, not merely the result. . . . Waiting to be happy limits our brain's potential for success, whereas cultivating positive brains makes us more motivated, efficient, resilient, creative, and productive, which drives performance upward.

Who knew all this time, through all our struggles, that our purpose was to seek happiness first and that the rest would follow?

Things won't make you happy for the long term. Other people won't make you happy long term, and neither will money. Even achievements won't make you happy long term. Sure, I understand the relief money provides, but it won't make you a happier person. Once the bills are paid, you'll be back to your old, familiar Emotional Age—your Dominant Emotional Archetype.

Give a spoiled child a new toy, and you'll understand immediately. More toys don't make the child a happier person; they may actually add fuel to her internal anger. Most children get overwhelmed with too much stuff. They don't need more things; kids need more love, acceptance, affection, compassion, tenderness, fun, empathy, joy, understanding, peaceful communication, and security—all the same things that we adults need!

Kids need to know they matter. They need to learn and witness healthy boundary setting. They need to feel safe and supported enough to dream big and then pursue those big dreams.

When this happens, children have a healthy sense of self-esteem, self-awareness, self-assertiveness, self-acceptance, self-confidence, self-love, and a level of joy. They know that no matter what, they can take care of themselves in the world.

Everything in our outer world is a reflection of our inner world—it reflects our level of trust, self-advocacy, and empowerment. When we are contracting, our life feels heavy and stressful, and we feel confused about our purpose. We don't feel safe, protected, and valuable. Life is hard, and work is exhausting. Money is scarce, clients are limited, and we're all in one big race—a competition of sorts—to reach the summit! *(And, it's lonely at the top.)*

When we are expansive, we feel hopeful, focused, and secure. We recognize our choices. We take calculated risks that, most often, pay off. We look forward to getting up each morning, excited about our possibilities. We know there is more than enough to go around. We are energized and motivated about our career and the work ahead of us.

*Does this mean that every single day of our lives is perfect and shiny?*

*No,* but more often than not, we feel content and at peace with things; we have the ability to look within to find our joy rather than allowing outside influences to steal our thunder, whether it's the weather, traffic, our mother-in-law, or our ex. We've taken control of our emotions. We're following our own inner light. We've set healthy boundaries with those who try to intrude on our dreams, desires, and purpose. We are expansive, empowered, unafraid!

## LIGHT YOUR FIRE

*Isn't it time to ask your Self, with a clear head and open eyes:* What lights my fire? What do I most want to feel, experience, become? What kind of legacy do I want to leave?

Now, I understand that you probably have a mortgage, a car payment, and/or a few mouths to feed, and that the notion of abandoning your day job in the hopes of playing baseball in the MLB or dancing on Broadway seems far-fetched. This is not what I'm suggesting. But passion is the oil for your internal fire; it's what creates the Light inside of you that nobody else can put out.

It reminds me of the little Sunday school song I learned as a child: "This little light of mine, I'm gonna let it shine!"

The Light is driven by your deepest desires (that you are not only permitted, but mandated, to pursue)! It is what expands collective consciousness!

You need to ask yourself what brings you the kind of passion that fills you with expansive joy, peace, and pleasure. It's time to allow yourself to enjoy what lights your inner fire. It's time to tell your Self the truth!

If you don't know the answers to these questions, don't fret. You aren't alone. Most people don't take the time to reflect on these most important questions. But happiness is a reflection of our self-awareness—of how closely we are aligned with our true authentic Self.

> **Your Light is flamed when you trust, listen to, and believe in your Self.**

Don't worry about which is the highest income-producing career, or if returning to school will leave you in debt for years. If it lights you up, move in that direction. If it drains your life force, move away. Trust your internal GPS—red light, yellow light, green light. And don't worry if going for the gusto feels overwhelming at first: start with small acts of courage.

When we get in the way of our passion, we are guaranteed tough times. When we follow our hearts, even if tough times come (and they will), we will have the energy, focus, and optimism to see them through. The truth will set us free! Follow your light like a beacon!

*How can you determine what creates light in your life?*

First and foremost, look at what you love to do for enjoyment! You will be amazed at the opportunities that come your way when you are open *and vocal* about your passions and desires.

As I mentioned in the Introduction, your desire is similar to a rocket firing upward from the surface of this earth. If your desires are powerful enough, there is nothing that will allow them to contract—or fail.

Be certain, however, to pursue only what you *really desire*, or you'll waste your time chasing things in vain. Gravity will pull you back down. You'll feel your life contracting. Instead, follow what lights you up—by doing so, *you'll feel enlightened!*

If you love singing and/or playing a musical instrument, stay open-minded when it comes to musical endeavors or opportunities. Maybe you aren't going to be a rock star, but you might discover or create a career that invites you to play, produce, or teach music to others—if you're open about your passion with yourself and with the people around you!

If you love reading or writing, make it a priority to do a little bit every day—all you need is a notebook and a library card. Today, it's incredibly easy to start a blog, share your opinions, and continue to develop your writing voice.

If you love sports and athletics, find a program specifically geared toward the body: physiotherapy, physical education, nutrition, personal training, even biology.

If you love supporting, inspiring, and motivating others, a career as an empowerment coach may be right up your alley. Or even event planning or public relations.

If you love debating or speaking in front of people, join Toastmasters—there are meet-up groups all over the world; or even consider becoming a lawyer, professor, or philosopher.

■

My youngest daughter has loved applying makeup and taking photos since she was a little girl. Now at nineteen, she's determined to be a special-effects makeup artist for Hollywood movies. Her photos are stunning. Her creativity is magnificent.

The funny thing is, she still hears from well-intending friends and family members that perhaps she should just do makeup for bridal parties since so few people ever make it to Hollywood. I remind her, "You'll always wonder *what if.* Don't sell your Self short. The world is your oyster."

My eldest daughter, on the other hand, struggled at first with finding her way. She would sometimes cry during her high school years, saying, "I don't know what I'm good at. I don't know what I should do for the rest of my life."

"You don't have to know what you're doing for the rest of your life!" I'd tell her. "Start by moving in the direction of what you are most interested in—the thing you secretly wish would happen but that you're afraid to verbalize to anyone. Don't worry about income. You can always make money once you do what you love. Don't worry about the *how.* Follow your *why.*"

**There is no "right" path.**
**But there is a "right path" for you!**

## YOUR CAREER STRATEGY

People often ask me how I have so much willpower to work the way I do. My response, "It takes willpower *not* to work. What I do for a living is not a job that I do begrudgingly. My work is my passion—it lights my fire!"

Some of my family members don't understand: "I don't care about your work. I don't want to hear about it," my brother has said to me on many occasions. "I want to know how *you* are doing and what *you* are up to!"

Well . . . if you ask me what's new, I'm going to tell you about my new book or about the retreat I'm holding at a gorgeous new location somewhere exciting in the world!

When you do what you love, your work *is* what's going on with you; you haven't compartmentalized yourself into "work life" and "real life." You are a whole being who is fully expressed in and enriched by the work that you do.

> When your work isn't your bliss, you'll have to fill your life up with a lot of things.

The great news is that you don't have to choose between having a job you don't enjoy but that comes with a good salary and pursuing a dream that excites you but that might not turn a profit. You can have both. You can love what you do and make enough money to pay for what you love. You can even have a wonderful love life, do what you love professionally, and make enough money to pay for it all! Yes, you can have it all.

If you need to make more money, there is always a way. You have to get into creative, expansive energy, though. Breathe! Let go of that fearful grip, and then be willing to look *and think* outside of the box. You have to first accept what is: take an honest reality check. And then focus on solutions rather than on the possibility of your failing.

Ask the right questions; don't let fear pull you back down. The answers are always there if you will allow yourself to become inspiring, innovative, and imaginative!

In my own career, I'm building a great company because I'm aware of my deepest desires—my purpose—and I'm constantly working on improving my communication skills to lead me to wherever I'm *really* meant to go. I'm healing the wounds that have kept me playing small and scared, I'm following my heart, and I'm attracting and working with other empowered people.

*(Listen up, Lone Wolf: You can't do it alone any longer!)*

You are only as successful as the people you spend the most amount of time with: birds of a feather flock together, so you have to be cognizant of those you are flocking with! Do your friends bring out the best in you? Does your family encourage you to expand your life? Are your coworkers themselves in pursuit of happiness, too?

If you don't feel like you are showing up as the greatest expression of your Self, go back to the chapter on Assertive Communication and master your communication skills—climb higher in your own personal empowerment! Expand your Emotional Edges!

Once you begin to expand into your happiness, you'll notice that you have more energy and you show up differently in the world. Your purpose will reveal itself, *almost naturally.* You won't have to pursue it the way you think you do: you'll work, but you will be your Real Self!

Once here, you will effortlessly begin to recognize *your career path* under one of the following three Dominant Career Strategies that I refer to as the Light Protector, the Light

Connector, and the Light Worker (notice this structure, too, is composed of three characters).

These three career strategies are, in essence, our "expanded" Parent and Child Emotional Sub-Archetypes; we have raised our level of communication and healed the wounds that previously robbed us of our power. We're following what lights us up, and we're trusting that all will work out.

Sure, we may still have the occasional setback and down day, but at this point, we know that suffering doesn't serve us. Instead, we see everything as signs leading us to greener pastures. We aren't following anyone else's desire. We trust ourselves—listening to and following our light.

When I refer to Light in terms of the Light Protector, the Light Connector, and the Light Worker, I'm describing energy.

I compare this energy to a dining room ceiling light with a dimmer switch: those of us who have expanded into the wholeness of our being resonate similarly to the full spectrum of light beaming throughout the room when the dimmer is set on high—we are bright and energized! We are full spectrum! We—literally—can lighten the mood wherever we go. We are tapped into Creative Energy. We feel good! People feel good being around us.

On the other hand, people who haven't identified the flaws in their communication habits or acknowledged the origins of their weaknesses and fears, or those who haven't embraced the gifts of their imperfections and learned from them—thus transcending their past—feel heavier or more oppressive to be around. They're still resonating in Passive, Passive-Aggressive, or Aggressive Communication strategies. They feel darker. The dimmer switch is dialed back to low.

*The interesting part is that science claims that we do actually emit light.* It isn't just New Age mumbo jumbo:

Dr. Fritz-Albert Popp, a German physicist and founder of the International Institute of Biophysics in Neuss, Germany, is credited with the discovery of biophoton emissions or tiny currents of light, or energy, emanating from all living things.

People can literally feel our Light when we walk into a room. It has nothing to do with the size or our hips, our bank account balance, or our achievements. It's the intensity of our energy.

Have you ever noticed how bright and lively some people's eyes are? And how the "soulless" seem to have eyes that are empty and dead?

Albert Einstein taught that energy and mass are perfectly interchangeable, and that very small amounts of mass may be converted into a very large amount of energy and vice versa. He explained it with $E = mc^2$:

> It followed from the special theory of relativity that mass and energy are both but different manifestations of the same thing—a somewhat unfamiliar conception for the average mind. Furthermore, the equation $E = mc^2$, in which energy is put equal to mass, multiplied by the square of the velocity of light, showed that very small amounts of mass may be converted into a very large amount of energy and vice versa.

This helps us understand that although we appear to be human beings, we are, in fact, beings of pure energy or light; some of us, as a result of our Emotional Age, are shining brighter than others. The more empowered we are, the brighter our light and the more able we are to see and make good choices. We have a greater perspective, more energy! We shine!

The important thing to remember when we are expanding our consciousness, or increasing the intensity of our light, is that we can't climb the Empowerment Spectrum without moving up one level at a time, the same way we can't turn a dimmer switch up without passing through every vibrational frequency. In other words, you can't jump from Passive to Peaceful Communication without experiencing all the levels in between. Yes—you have to face and feel your anger and you must authentically forgive; you must own all of yourself to shine in high-definition.

Once we have moved up the Empowerment Spectrum, we will feel ourselves shifting to this new, lighter, more empowered way of engaging with the world, a way that is filled with love and passion and understanding.

**Creative Energy is the most powerful force in the Universe.**

This takes mindfulness. We must ask ourselves throughout the day: "Am I feeling expansive or contracted? Breathing deeply or shallowly? Open-minded or close-minded? Fearless or gripping? What would I need to *let go of* in order to feel lighter?"

Let's now look at the three Dominant Career Strategies in more detail. As you read each description, you will naturally feel more connected to one. Be aware that similarly to the Three Dominant Archetypes, we each embody all three of these career strategies but most often one is more dominant: the Light Protector, the Light Connector, or the Light Worker.

*The following section is intended to provide you with a guide to help you source out a career that you most resonate with . . .*

## THE LIGHT PROTECTOR

The Light Protectors are protectors of the Light! They have mastered the balancing act of give and take. And although they give *of* themselves, true Light Protectors don't give *up* themselves. Often referred to as the "salt of the earth," you can count on these people. They have strength, conviction, integrity, and accountability. If a Light Protector offers to help you, you're in good hands! Most often, these people are the expanded Parent Archetype.

Light Protectors are never bullies or persecutors, and they have no tolerance for violence or exploitation. These are many of our unsung (s)heroes: doctors, firefighters, police officers, nurses, paramedics, detectives, judges, prosecutors, producers, publishers, naturopaths, scientists, those in research and development, photographers, videographers, environmentalists, pilots, dentists, editors, volunteers, advocates, executive assistants, accountants, principals, managers, chief operations officers, coaches, therapists, psychiatrists, chiropractors, trainers, farmers, health-care providers, lawyers, librarians, and so on.

Caretaking, protecting, and nurturing come naturally to the Light Protectors, but they are not martyrs, victims, or rescuers to anyone.

## THE LIGHT CONNECTOR

The Light Connectors, on the other hand, are the ultra networkers—the social butterflies. They love spreading the Light! They, too, have expanded or transcended their disempowered Emotional Sub-Archetypes and are excited about sharing people, products, services, and/or causes they love!

The Light Connectors are always joining or attending conferences, meetings, events, groups, social/business dates, etc. They know "who's who," what's trending, and what's cutting edge. And if they love you, they will tell the world! These people need to be in the action. Life is all about connecting the dots. With a business card, smartphone, and extensive contact list at their fingertips, they do their best work: *"You need to meet so and so! I'm not sure why, but I think the two of you could do amazing things together!"*

The Light Connectors don't necessarily write the books or invent the products but when they love something, they'll share it as though it's their own. Event organizers, salespeople, brokers, bloggers, philanthropists, fund-raisers, real estate agents, flight attendants, social media experts, servers, agents, managers, promoters, supporters, coordinators, publicists, and marketing executives are the Light Connectors of the world.

Remember, being a Light Connector is different from simply being a networker. Light Connectors have expanded their Emotional Edge and are using their great energy and outgoing personalities to expand the Light—to expand consciousness!

## THE LIGHT WORKER

Edith Wharton broke through limits of late-nineteenth, early twentieth-century society to become one of America's greatest writers—and this at a time when women had no rights. She explains the Light Worker's purpose in this way: *"There are two ways of spreading light: to be the candle or the mirror that reflects it."* The Light Worker is the candle!

Light Workers love to be up front and center—expanding consciousness and spreading the Light! They thrive in the spotlight. They aren't seeking attention, they're following their calling. The bigger the crowd, the greater they shine! The Light Worker is a conduit of consciousness, allowing Creative Energy to flow through them. They may be shy or quiet in their personal lives (although, not necessarily) but once they step onto the stage, so to speak, they and the collective consciousness—the Light—expands. They are passionate about "waking people up!" They shine brightly!

The Light Workers are our artists, actors, singers, musi-
cians, comedians, writers, journalists, directors, professors,
motivational speakers, spokespeople, teachers, clergy, politi-
cians, designers, carpenters, chefs, stylists, creative directors,
dancers, radio or TV hosts, chief executive officers, even professional athletes—people comfortable standing up and standing out.

Similar to both the Light Protectors and the Light Connectors, the Light Workers have done the work, have healed the
wounds, and they are ready and willing to share their Light—
liberating others to shine brightly, too!

■

In my business, I'm mindful to employ members of all three of
these Dominant Career Strategies on my upper-level manage-
ment team. For instance, having too many Light Protectors
and not enough Light Connectors means the work won't get
out to the world, no matter how good it is. Too many Light
Connectors can lead to a situation where nobody is actually
doing the work, even though the organization has a great repu-
tation for being filled with passionate, energetic people. And
too many Light Workers is like having too many chefs in the
kitchen. They don't mean to, but they can "spoil the broth"
when they're all dug into their own vision for the best way to
execute a plan. If not reined in, their energy is just too intense
for them to spend time together effectively. As an example, just
look at how many Hollywood couples stay married. If Light
Workers don't learn how to manage their own light, they can
overwhelm and "flood" each other.

If you own a company that's struggling, even though you
employ top-notch staff, pay attention to their personal career
strategies to determine if you have the right people in the right

spots in your business, or as bestselling author and business strategist Jim Collins refers to it: "in your bus." He points out in *Good to Great*:

> When we began the research project, we expected to find that the first step in taking a company from good to great would be to set a new direction, a new vision and strategy for the company, and then to get people committed and aligned behind the new direction.
>
> We found something quite the opposite.
>
> The executives who ignited the transformation from good to great did not first figure out where to drive the bus and then get people to take it there. No, they first got the right people on the bus (and the wrong people off the bus) and then figured out where to drive it. They said, in essence, "Look, I don't really know where we should take the bus. But I know this much: If we get the right people on the bus, the right people in the right seats, and the wrong people off the bus, then we'll figure out how to take it someplace great."

Your dream will never fully manifest until you align with the right people, who each embrace their natural-born tendencies. In other words, you need to get the right people in the right seats in your business. This allows us to bring out the best in one another!

Be cognizant in your own life—both professional and personal—with who you are surrounding yourself with.

If you are a Light Worker, you will naturally find yourself being attracted toward Light Protectors—people who help you stay strong, inspired, and healthy; and even if they overprotect from time to time, at least you'll understand now why you've chosen the Protectors you have!

You will also find Light Connectors who are skilled and passionate about sharing your gifts and talents with others. Embrace them! True Light Connectors will never be jealous of you; they are driven to connect the dots and make things happen!

If you are a Light Protector, it's normal for you to find yourself attracted to those who embody the other two career strategies—the Light Workers and the Light Connectors. You are naturally driven to serve and protect.

And for the Light Connectors—you, too, need to balance your relationships and surround yourselves with some individuals who expand and excite you as well as those who keep you grounded. You'll notice that the best collaborations are when there is a trinity of these three Dominant Career Strategies.

## No More Contracting

If the idea of having your own book published secretly makes you giddy, or playing your music to large stadiums of adoring fans excites you (Light Workers), if traveling to the deep seas of Greenland as a marine biologist keeps you awake at night, or opening your own safe haven to help protect women and children lights your fire (Light Protectors); if being on the ground floor of the New York Stock Exchange or "hobnobbing" with socialites gives you butterflies (Light Connectors), *why aren't you pursuing these dreams?*

Most likely, it's because you haven't yet expanded your energy and risen into the higher levels of consciousness or communication. *But you are on your way!*

If you have been navigating your life as the Parent Archetype, you've most likely had a hard time protecting yourself, even though you seem to protect everyone else. Perhaps, you struggle charging the right fees for what you're worth; maybe you feel as though you should be volunteering or you think that rich people must somehow be ripping others off.

If you have been resonating as the Child Archetype, there's a good chance you've been waiting for someone to come along and notice you. No wonder you need so much attention! You desperately want to be "somebody" but you still aren't sure how to dig in, apply the lessons, and create the success you so deserve!

The great news is that *now that you know* how to expand and rise into your most empowered Adult Self by "healing the split," you will be able to have a career that you love and income to help you enjoy all of life's greatest pleasures!

Now don't get me wrong: doing what you love doesn't mean you won't, perhaps, put in long hours and miss time at home occasionally. There is no "perfect" position. Even the greatest jobs have downfalls. The secret is getting clear about what you're good at, what comes naturally, and what lights your inner fire. Follow the Light!

You know the rules now, if you want to feel empowered:

1. Think for yourself and make choices that feel right for you.
2. Catch yourself when you're sabotaging, or contracting into fear. Stop and take a deep breath.
3. Ask yourself: "What Dominant Emotional Archetype am I behaving in? Which archetype would I rather be in? What would courage have me do?"

Let's look finally at how the Three Dominant Archetypes show up with work and money.

## Career, Money, and the Parent Archetype

The term *Imposter Syndrome* was first coined by clinical psychologists Pauline R. Clance and Suzanne A. Imes in 1978 when they observed many high-achieving females who believed they were not intelligent and were overevaluated by others.

Jenna Goudreau wrote a compelling article in *Forbes* magazine that showcased women such as Sheryl Sandberg, Sonia Sotomayor, Meryl Streep, and Tina Fey, who each feared they didn't deserve their accomplishments and considered themselves frauds.

Doesn't that sound crazy? How can these wildly successful and brilliant women look at what they've accomplished and not believe in themselves?

Or maybe it sounds familiar to you? *Especially if you've been navigating in the Parent Archetype!*

I remember feeling this same way myself when I received my first book deal with Hay House Publishing in 2003. I was having lunch with the president when I confessed, "I'm afraid I might not be qualified enough to share the stage with Louise Hay or Dr. Wayne Dyer. I'm not sure if I should have my own radio show with Hay House Radio and Sirius Satellite." He chuckled and told me I was suffering from Imposter Syndrome.

Many of the most successful people in the world have worried that someone is going to discover they aren't good enough. These are, almost without exception, people who embody the Parent Archetype—the Martyr, the Rescuer, the Puritan, the Busy Bee, the Perfectionist, the Micromanager, and the Ruler are all perfect examples!

According to long-time lecturer and leading author on the phenomenon of the Imposter Syndrome, Valerie Young, EdD, little has changed in the last three decades—except that more women are susceptible to this syndrome:

> Always waiting for the other shoe to drop. You feel as if you've flown
> under the radar, been lucky, or that they just like you. If you dismiss

your accomplishments and abilities, you're left with one conclusion:
That you've fooled them.

Do you get it? You are not alone. Many people who achieve more than they dreamed they ever could are afraid they aren't enough *when they are*!

This is when the whole "fake it till you make it" comes into play. Forget about the fear and follow your bliss. Expand your horizons! To make changes, all it takes is mindfulness and self-awareness.

Ask yourself: "If I felt more empowered in my career, I would _____ (fill in the blank). If money, time, and responsibilities were no object, I would _____ (fill in the blank)."

It's time for you to rise from being the wind beneath everyone else's wings; it's time for you to fly! Be the Light Worker, the Light Connector, or the Light Protector you've always wanted to be! It's your time!

## Career, Money, and the Child Archetype

The Child Archetype struggles with money and career more than any of the other archetypes. They have a hard time keeping a job or staying committed to a career path. There is always drama that distracts them from fulfilling their dreams and purpose. They often arrive late or leave early; perhaps they don't get along with a coworker, or their boss is always picking on them. Something is always wrong.

Along with workplace struggles, those who embody the Child Archetype usually have finances that are a mess. Maybe their credit is bad, their taxes are in arrears, they've borrowed money they can't pay back, or they are dependent on another person to pay their way. Their excuses are countless.

The Child Archetype has some serious growing up to do if they want abundance and prosperity—along with a career that they love! They simply struggle with their commitments, not realizing the recognition that comes from long-time effort rather than short-term bursts of attention.

If this sounds like you, it's important to be patient, to work hard, to be diligent, and to set your sights on executing big-picture goals rather than nipping at very short-term projects that don't pay off. Above all, focus on expanding your Emotional Edge! As my brother once told me many years ago, "Focus on the deal, not on the dollar." This means you shouldn't get caught up in short-term, get-rich-quick schemes or "plowing through" one job after another in search of gold. The payoff will come when you invest your time and commitment into building solid projects and relationships, based on integrity, quality, and dedication.

If you were to spend a day with the most successful person you know, you'd see that he or she is consistent and steady—"minoring in majors" as they say, rather than "majoring in minors." Successful people are able to distinguish between being productive and being busy.

The truth is, when it comes to money, slow and steady wins the race every time. When it comes to building your dreams, it is the daily, seemingly insignificant choices you make that will determine how your retirement package looks!

Patience is a virtue, one that the Child Archetype can and must learn! The great news is that if they do . . . if they expand their Emotional Edge . . . these people can become incredible Light Workers, Light Protectors, or Light Connectors, as well!

# Career, Money, and the Adult Archetype

The Adult Archetype follows his or her heart, especially when it comes to a career. They get involved in few power struggles, which makes working with them a joy. If those who navigate in the Adult Archetype are self-employed, they understand their client's needs and can speak to their demographic, presenting themselves with confidence, ease, and grace. They are solution-oriented team players, having the courage to both lead and listen. Drama is absent from their workplace demeanor, as they focus on getting the job done with joy, excellence, and commitment.

Although they arrive on time and put in a full day, these people know they aren't Superwoman or Superman and won't take on more than they can afford to lose. Those around the Adult are amazed at their energy, patience, willingness, and ambition. They are movers and shakers. Assertive, confident, and composed.

These are where we find the Light Workers, Light Protectors, and Light Connectors. These people are shifting the collective consciousness just by being themselves and living their lives with such authenticity, honesty, excitement, and joy!

This is the quest for all of us!

# Wake Up, World

Just as there are the Light Workers, the Light Protectors, and the Light Connectors, there are those who perpetrate fear and darkness in this world. Instead of spreading light, they try to steal our power from us.

Some call them soulless, heartless, even evil. Bullies. Perpetrators. They are the wolves—*sometimes but not always*—in sheep's clothing. They are part of what I call the Machine. (I know this is a topic most of us want to avoid.)

The Machine knows exactly what it wants: greed, gluttony, and materialism. And it will do whatever it has to do in order to win, i.e., "its desires outweigh your needs."

The Machine depends upon the masses to stay asleep so they won't notice all the carnage committed in the name of profit—including starvation, poverty, war, oppression, and abuse. The Machine rules the smallest infractions as well as the largest exploitations—from the thug who robs us of our last few dollars, to the rapist who robs us of our personal safety and innocence, to the murderer who robs us of our life, to corrupt corporations that enslave and exploit children, women, men, animals, and the earth, all in the name of money.

The Sheeple are those I half-jokingly refer to as people who are disempowered and disconnected from the bigger picture; distracted, out of the flow, and unaware, they are too consumed with their own struggles to pay attention to the collective consciousness. They are unconsciously giving away their power.

I don't mean to insult or sound callous when I use the term *Sheeple*; it's my way of pointing out how lost and alone so many people are, and how desperately they need to find a Shepherd to lead them back toward the Light—toward their own power!

Many Sheeple want to be Shepherds, but they're afraid: "*You* can't make a significant difference in this world!" they've been told. "Who do you think *you* are? Stay out of it! It's not your business. Focus on your own problems!"

Fear teaches us that we must dehumanize others in order for us to stay safe. We create separation and borders. Curfews and rules. Good and bad. Us against them. Us against ourselves.

Oh . . . and yes, they are taught the same things as we are:

Ominous, looming attacks dominant their dinner conversations, too.

The only way we can help heal this world is by having the Emotional Edge—to be wise with our choices and to use Assertive Communication and higher to evoke change. We must never allow fear to scare us into running away, burying our head in the sand, or staying silent. We must become Shepherds: Light Workers, Light Protectors, and Light Connectors!

*What about you?* Do you know what is happening outside of your neck of the woods—the atrocities being committed against *your* fellow human beings? Do you have any idea how many people are dying unnecessarily every day around the world? And are you doing anything to help those who are oppressed—those who have a voice but can't use it?

In 2014, we witnessed the ALS Ice Bucket Challenge sweep the globe. In roughly thirty days, over a hundred million dollars was raised for research and development for ALS, or Lou Gehrig's disease. Who knew that individuals worldwide filming themselves dump a bucket of icy water over their heads could raise this much money? It showed us the power that we—the masses—have when we splash a little cold water in our faces and wake up!

> The fact is, everyone deserves to have food in their belly, a safe place to lay their head at night, and the choice to expand their lives—it's not just an American dream.

Together, we can change things! If enough empowered people speak up and speak out, we will shift the tipping point!

As Glinda the Good Witch told Dorothy, "You've always had the power."

*So have you!*

Dorothy's power didn't come from that scared little man with a booming voice who was hiding behind a curtain, claiming to be the Almighty Wizard; nor did it come from wearing ruby-red slippers or clicking her heels three times (although, once again, the number three is powerful). The Scarecrow's brain did not come from a rolled-up diploma, the Cowardly Lion's courage from a medal of valor, or the Tin Man's heart from a large dangling red, heart-shaped clock. It came from deciding to stop following the yellow brick road and to stop believing someone else had the answers for them. It came from discovering they'd been navigating their lives as disempowered Emotional Sub-Archetypes based on what others told them they could or couldn't be. Their individual empowerments came from waking up and believing in themselves.

Once more I'm reminded of the fabulous movie *The Matrix*. (This film clearly had a massive impact on me!) If you saw it, you'll never forget the scene in which Laurence Fishburne, who plays a father figure, the godlike character called Morpheus, tells Neo—the chosen one (or chosen son)—played by Keanu Reeves:

> You take the blue pill, the story ends. You wake up in your bed and believe whatever you want to believe. You take the red pill, you stay in wonderland, and I show you how deep the rabbit hole goes.

This book is offering you the red pill . . . but the Machine will try to convince you to swallow the blue one. In fact, it's shocking that while handing us the *blue pill*, along with a list of its horrendous consequences, the Machine is able to promise such a great emotional payoff that we will happily swallow it anyway.

One may pose the question: Can the Light be turned on for *everyone*? Can we wake the Sheeple? And can we pull the invisible plug on the Machine?

The answer is absolutely!

The world is waking up!

Can you feel it?

■

As this chapter comes to a close, I'm sure you feel yourself expanding already! We live in an ever-expanding, infinite universe and you are a part of that universe. Your purpose is to become the most empowered version of you possible, and that means following your passions!

Stay focused on your desires—those rockets firing upward from the surface of this earth. If you don't really want something, don't give power to it. Stick with what lights you up, and you won't fail. Trust your inner GPS. It is a global positioning system. Literally.

Looking back at my personal empowerment journey that began almost twenty years ago with my first-ever journal and the first sentence I wrote: *"I just want to be empowered,"* I've done a lot of healing. My heart feels *nearly* whole. I'm in a much better place now. Not because I'm thinner, wealthier, sexier, or even smarter than I was back then: *I'm happier.* I'm constantly expanding my Emotional Edges. I'm done with suffering. This new space feels good. Freeing. Safe. Joyous. Exciting. Empowered. Yes, I'm certain this is what joy feels like.

To both my male and female readers, I hope that after reading this book the word *woman* signifies empowerment to you: love, joy, and peace.

We women are going to help heal the world. In the words

of John Lennon: "You may say that I'm a dreamer, but I'm not the only one. I hope someday you'll join us. And the world will live as one." Let's #CloseTheGap faster.

Thank you for taking this journey with me.

The world is waiting for you.

Be your Self!

# Acknowledgments

Leah Miller, my editor—you helped me find my Truth. Thank you for your thought-provoking questions, suggestions, and gentle criticisms that expanded my consciousness, pushed me out of my comfort zone, and helped me articulate *The Emotional Edge*. I am forever grateful to you!

Izabela Viskupova—your brilliant brain, adventurous spirit, and willing heart have been huge gifts to me—*and to this book*. Your excellent research and development helped me immensely. Your commitment to the Truth, your dedication to The S.W.A.T. Institute, and your compassion for the world are mind-blowing. I am so blessed to know you and work with you. Thank you for all you've done for *The Emotional Edge*!

Jen Taylor—what a stellar job you've done helping me to write and refine the Emotional Sub-Archetypes! I know we both felt like Mad Scientists at times—working around the clock, writing feverishly until all hours of the night! Your Creative Energy is magnificent, and your beautiful heart and mind are just that: beautiful! Thank you for your love and support over the years!

Heather Jackson, Tina Constable, and the rest of the amazing team at Harmony Books—thank you for helping me share my light with the world. I am so grateful to you and your expertise. Fingers crossed—I think we've "done good" with this one!

Colette Baron-Reid—the first words you spoke to me nearly fifteen years ago were *"Your work is going to help heal the world!"* I didn't know how to receive that fully then, but your belief in me, over the years, has kept me going through some of my darkest hours. Thank you for all that you are, for who you are, and for how you show up so courageously in this world. I love you. I believe you.

Yvonne MacRae—witnessing the birth and growth of our school has been the most monumental experience for me both personally and professionally. Without you and your wisdom, hard work, and strength, we could not have built this global coalition that is changing lives and empowering women. I love you!

Natalie Hughes—Thirty-five years of friendship, love, support, purpose, passion, and dreaming! *Oh my sister. It is time. Stand up.* Are you ready to rock the world with me?

Chantale Bondoux—Thank you for your never-ending support. You are my sister from another mister and I am so thankful that I can count on you no matter what, no matter when, no matter how. I love you!

Yvette Murray—thank you for your endless energy, positive attitude, enduring patience, and beautiful soul. You've been such a wonderful Light Protector and Light Connector for both The S.W.A.T. Institute and for me—both personally and professionally. On behalf of our entire team, thank you for all that you do and for how you show up in the world. You rock!

To the entire staff at The S.W.A.T. Institute—thank you for your dedication to the expansion of women's empowerment! You are doing such an amazing job! The world is a better place because of you!

To my students—thanks for teaching me so much; through listening, sharing, talking, coaching, crying, and reading your words, I am transformed.

David Nelson—having you at the stern has given me the faith and confidence to sail some rocky seas. You're a wonderful agent and an even greater human being. Thank you for believing in me.

Kamen Nikolov—you've watched, helped, and supported my professional growth for nearly fifteen years. You are a Creative Genius and a Light Protector of the highest caliber! Thank you for all your designs, Web sites, book covers, and so on. You get me. You get the movement. And for that I am so grateful.

My God—the Father, the Son, and the Holy Ghost; the Mother, the Daughter, and the Holy Spirit; the Selfless, the Selfish, and the Self. Amen and amen. The *wholly* trinity is my religion.

Oh, and to Florence + The Machine, Coldplay, and Lana Del Rey—You expanded my edges and lifted me higher. I listened to you day in and day out, earphones on, music pumping, throughout this entire writing process. Thank you for your courage, brilliance, and beauty. You expand the Light in a massive way!

Last but not least, to my children, Madelaine and Julia— Believe in love. It moves mountains. Believe in yourself.

You'll move mountains. And to my husband, Aaron James Morissette—thank you for "seeing" me the minute you met me. Really seeing me. Your love has helped me heal mountains of wounds. I love you. Thank you for all your support! Let's rock it, baby!

Breathe.

# Notes

**INTRODUCTION**

7   **The discovery that the universe:** Stephen Hawking, *A Brief History of Time* (New York: Bantam Books, 1988).

11   **Women are persons in matters:** Vivien Hughes, "How the Famous Five in Canada Won Personhood for Women," *London Journal of Canadian Studies* (2001–2002), http://www.canadian-studies.net/lccs/LJCS/Vol_17/Hughes.pdf.

13   **It's been a long, slow:** Caitlin Moran, *How to Be a Woman* (New York: Harper Perennial, 2011).

14   **The Wise Old Woman:** Carl Jung, *Man and His Symbols*, 2nd edition (London: Aldus, 1972).

**CHAPTER 1: YOUR EMOTIONAL AGE**

22   **Each person decides in early:** Eric Berne, *What Do You Say After You Say Hello?* (London: Corgi Books, 1975).

23   **Cognitive neuroscientist Michael Gazzaniga:** Michael Gazzaniga, *The Cognitive Neurosciences III*, 3rd revised edition (Cambridge, MA: MIT Press, 2004).

23   **The brain is a belief:** Michael Shermer, *The Believing Brain* (New York: Times Books, 2011).

24   **In a way, your "story":** Michael Gazzaniga, *The Cognitive Neurosciences III*.

28  **Infants, almost as if they:** Muriel James and Dorothy
Jongeward, *Born to Win*, Twenty-fifth anniversary edition
(Cambridge: Da Capo, 1996).

28  **Children's first feelings about themselves:** Ibid.


## CHAPTER 2: THREE DOMINANT ARCHETYPES

46  **I have long believed that:** Caroline Myss, *Archetypes: Who
Are You?* (Carlsbad, CA: Hay House, 2013).

47  **The "superego" which plays:** John Maltby, Liz Day, and
Ann Macaskill, *Personality, Individual Differences, and Intelligence*
(Essex, England: Pearson, 2013).

47  **The "ego," also known as the Self:** John Maltby, Liz
Day, and Ann Macaskill, *Personality, Individual Differences, and
Intelligence* (Essex, England: Pearson, 2013).

47  **Jung acknowledged Freud's theory:** Daniel Cervone and
Lawrence Pervin, *Personality: Theory and Research*, 12th edition (Hoboken, NJ: Wiley, 2013).

48  **At any given moment each:** Eric Berne, *Games People Play*
(New York: Penguin, 1987).

92  **"There is nothing more important":** Michael A. Singer,
*The Untethered Soul: The Journey Beyond Yourself* (Oakland,
CA: New Harbinger Publications and Noetic Books, 2007).

92  **"True personal growth is about transcending":** Ibid.


## CHAPTER 3: THE COMMUNICATION SCALE

102  **"learned helplessness":** Henry Gleitman, *Psychology*, 6th
revised edition (New York: W. W. Norton, 2004).

104  **"Did I cause this?":** Ibid.

109  **Come to the edge:** Christopher Logue, *New Numbers* (London: Jonathan Cape, 1969).

124  **Humans appear to fear similar things:** David Ropeik,
"The Consequences of Fear," supplement, *European Molecular
Biology Organization Report* (Oct. 5, 2004): S56–S59, http://
www.ncbi.nlm.nih.gov/pmc/articles/PMC1299209/.

124  **In the United States alone:** David Ropeik, "The

Consequences of Fear," supplement, *European Molecular Biology Organization Report* (Oct. 5, 2004): S56–S59, http://www.ncbi.nlm.nih.gov/pmc/articles/PMC1299209/.

126    **There were few animals killed:** Benjamin Radford, "Tsunamis and Animal 'Sixth Sense' Warnings." Discovery Communications, 2011, http://news.discovery.com/animals/pets/tsunamis-and-animal-sixth-sense-warnings-110311.htm.

133    **Sometimes unresolved guilt and shame:** Melody Beattie, *Finding Your Way Home* (New York: Harper Collins, 1998).

134    **Sigmund Freud's daughter, Anna:** Anna Freud, *The Ego and the Mechanisms of Defense* (London: Hogarth Press and Institute of Psycho-Analysis, 1937).

134    **Sooner or later, we must all:** Iyanla Vanzant, *In the Meantime* (New York: Fireside, 1998).


### CHAPTER 4: EMPOWERED COMMUNICATION BEGINS

146    **When an assertive person interacts:** Robert Alberti and Michael Emmons, *Your Perfect Right: Assertiveness and Equality in Your Life and Relationships*, 9th revised edition (Atascadero, CA: Impact Publishers, 2008).

146    **The first and basic act:** Nathaniel Branden, *The Six Pillars of Self-Esteem* (New York: Bantam Books, 1995).

147    **"It is a discipline whereby you maintain":** Lynne McTaggart, *The Intention Experiment* (New York: Atria, 2007).

148    **From kindergarten on, the focus:** Ellen J. Langer, *Mindfulness* (Cambridge: Da Capo, 1989.) Print.

151    **Spiritual teacher Byron Katie:** Byron Katie, *Loving What Is: Four Questions That Can Change Your Life* (New York: Harmony Books, 2002).

183    **Just watch a sunset:** Fraser Cain, "How Fast Does the Earth Rotate?" *Universe Today*, May 20, 2013, http://www.universetoday.com/26623/how-fast-does-the-earth-rotate/#ixzz34FWSxveZ.

184    **"At this level" he says:** David Hawkins, *Power vs. Force* (Carlsbad, CA: Hay House, 1995).

## CHAPTER 5: WHO AM I?

192   **Healing the split requires us:** Debbie Ford, *Why Good People Do Bad Things: How to Stop Being Your Own Worst Enemy* (New York: HarperCollins, 2008).

195   **This aspect of you only appears:** Marianne Williamson, *A Course in Weight Loss: 21 Spiritual Lessons for Surrendering Your Weight Forever* (Carlsbad, CA: Hay House, 2010).

217   **In fact, science confirms that the brains of people:** M. F. O'Connor, D. K. Wellisch, A. L. Stanton, N. I. Eisenberger, M. R. Irwin, and M. D. Lieberman, "Craving Love? Enduring Grief Activates Brain's Reward Center," *Neuroimage* 42, no. 2 (Aug. 15, 2008): 969–72.


## CHAPTER 6: CONDUIT OF CONSCIOUSNESS

223   **A woman's relationship with her:** Sarah Ban Breathnach, *Simple Abundance: A Daybook of Comfort and Joy* (New York: Warner Books, 1995).

227   **Worldwide there is a rising incidence:** Chester Alper, "Polygenic Diseases on the Rise." Immune Disease Institute, Harvard Medical School, 2004–2014, http://www.idi.harvard .edu/news_events/articles/polygenic_diseases_on_the_rise/.

227   **You can't hurt a part of the whole:** Eric Stice and Sonja Spoor, "Relation of Reward from Food Intake and Anticipated Food Intake to Obesity: A Functional Magnetic Resonance Imaging Study." National Center for Biotechnology Information, 2009, http://www.ncbi.nlm.nih.gov/pmc/ articles/PMC2681092/.

229   **"In order for man to succeed":** John J. Ratey, *Spark* (New York: Little Brown and Company, 2008).

230   **It turns out that neuroscientists:** Ibid.

230   **"Exercise," Ratey says:** Ibid.

230   **In today's technology-driven:** Ibid.

232   **The great news is that finally:** Ibid.

232   **Note: It's hard to believe:** Ibid.

232   **There are many theories:** "Why Do We Sleep, Anyway?"

Healthy Sleep, the Division of Sleep Medicine at Harvard
Medical School, 2007, http://healthysleep.med.harvard.edu/
healthy/matters/benefits-of-sleep/why-do-we-sleep.

233   **The average adult requires:** Crystal Andrus, *Simply . . .
Woman! The 12-Week Body-Mind-Soul Total Transformation Program* (Carlsbad, CA: Hay House, 2004).

234   **"Humor, games, roughhousing, flirtation":** Stuart
Brown, *Play Is More Than Just Fun*. Filmed May 2008 at Serious Play. Ted Talk: http://www.ted.com/talks/stuart_brown
_says_play_is_more_than_fun_it_s_vital?language=en.

236   **Brown has spent decades studying:** Margarita Tartakovsky, "The Importance of Play for Adults," Psych Central,
http://psychcentral.com/blog/archives/2012/11/15/the
-importance-of-play-for-adults/.

236   **A recent study conducted by scientists:** Lecia Buschak,
"Benefits of Ecotherapy: Being in Nature Fights Depression,
Improves Mental Health and Well-Being," *Healthy Living*
(Oct. 26, 2013), http://www.medicaldaily.com/benefits
-ecotherapy-being-nature-fights-depression-improves-mental
-health-and-well-being-261075.

237   **Being in nature has been proven:** "New Research Shows
Benefits of Ecotherapy for Mental Health and Wellbeing,"
*Mind* (Oct. 23, 2013), http://www.mind.org.uk/news
-campaigns/news/new-research-shows-benefits-of
-ecotherapy-for-mental-health-and-wellbeing/
#.VEWF5IfldKo.

237   **By tapping into the restorative powers:** Richard Louv,
*The Nature Principle: Reconnecting with Life in a Virtual Age*
(Chapel Hill, NC: Algonquin Books, 2012).


**CHAPTER 7: WHO ARE YOU?**

258   **Women have a larger behavioral repertoire:** Melissa
Kaplan, "UCLA Study on Friendship Among Women,"
*Chronic Neuroimmune Diseases* (2014), http://www.anapsid.org/
cnd/gender/tendfend.html.

260    **It is also interesting to note:** Mona Lisa Schulz, MD, PhD, *The New Feminine Brain: How Women Can Develop Their Inner Strengths, Genius, and Intuition* (New York: Free Press, 2005).

260    **"The Four Horsemen of the Apocalypse":** John Gottman, PhD, *Why Marriages Succeed or Fail: And How You Can Make Yours Last* (New York: Simon & Schuster, 1994).

262    **Almost 40 percent of women:** John Gray, *Venus on Fire, Mars on Ice: Hormonal Balance—The Key to Life, Love and Energy* (Coquitlam, BC: Mind Publishing, 2012).

262    **When I talk about the enormous stress:** Ibid.

263    **The average forty-year-old man:** Ibid.

263    **From diabetes, depression, high blood pressure**: Matt MacMillen, "Low Testosterone: How Do You Know When Levels Are Too Low?" *Men's Health*, http://www.webmd.com/men/features/low-testosterone-explained-how-do-you-know-when-levels-are-too-low.

267    **"This calls to mind a story":** Crystal Andrus, *Transcendent Beauty* (Carlsbad, CA: Hay House, 2006).

271    **There is a mysterious, indescribable:** Rob Bell, *The Zimzum of Love: A New Way of Understanding Marriage* (New York: HarperOne, 2014).

274    **"People speak different love languages":** Gary Chapman, *The 5 Love Languages: The Secret to Love That Lasts* (Chicago: Northfield Publishing, 1992).

275    **To be in alignment with "what is":** Eckhart Tolle, *A New Earth* (New York: Penguin, 2005).

275    **It is the Presence:** David Hawkins, *Power vs. Force* (Carlsbad, CA: Hay House, 1995).

278    **When you first met your lover:** Laura Berman, *Real Sex for Real Women* (New York: Dorling Kindersley, 2010).

## CHAPTER 8: WHAT'S MY PURPOSE?

284    **More than a decade of groundbreaking research:** Shawn Achor, *The Happiness Advantage* (New York: Crown Business, 2010).

292 **Dr. Fritz-Albert Popp, a German physicist:** Fritz-Albert Popp, "International Institute of Biophysics," http://www .biontology.com/international-institute-of-biophysics/.

292 **It followed from the special theory:** Max Born, *Atomic Physics*, 8th edition (New York: Dover Publications, 1989).

297 **When we began the research project:** Jim Collins, *Good to Great* (New York: HarperCollins, 2001).

300 **Jenna Goudreau wrote a compelling article:** Jenna Goudreau, "When Women Feel Like Frauds They Fuel Their Own Failures," *Forbes*, October 19, 2011, http://www.forbes .com/sites/jennagoudreau/2011/10/19/women-feel-like -frauds-failures-tina-fey-sheryl-sandberg/.

300 **Always waiting for the other shoe:** Valerie Young, *The Secret Thoughts of Successful Women* (New York: Crown Business, 2011).

# Index

## ABOUT THE AUTHOR

**CRYSTAL ANDRUS MORISSETTE** is a worldwide leader in the field of self-discovery and transformation. After overcoming insurmountable odds, Crystal has risen to become a women's advocate, bestselling author, beloved Master Empowerment Coach, international speaker, TV personality, and founder of The S.W.A.T. Institute (Simply Woman Accredited Trainer), an international Empowerment Coaching Certification school exclusively for women.

Certified by the American College of Sports Medicine and Canadian School of Natural Nutrition, Crystal has shared the stage with some of the world's top "movers and shakers," including Dr. Phil, Dr. Wayne Dyer, Suze Orman, Louise Hay, Naomi Judd, and Sarah Ferguson, the Duchess of York, just to name a few. Crystal lives in a small town in Ontario, Canada, with her husband, two daughters, four furry friends, and a flock of singing canaries!

To enroll in her 12-Week TeleCourse: The Emotional Edge or to become a Master Empowerment Coach, please visit www.SWATinstitute.com.